Tests of Voice, Speech and Language

Tests of Voice, Speech and Language

Edited by Myra Kersner, MSc, DipCSLT, DipDrTh

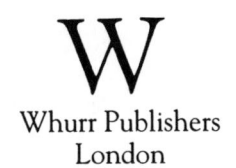

Whurr Publishers
London

© Myra Kersner 1992

First published 1992 by
Whurr Publishers Ltd
19B Compton Terrace, London N1 2UN, England

All rights reserved. No part of this publication may be reproduced, stored in a retrieval system, or transmitted in any form or by any means, electronic, mechanical, photocopying, recording or otherwise, without the prior permission of Whurr Publishers Limited.

This publication is sold subject to the conditions that it shall not, by way of trade or otherwise, be lent, resold, hired out, or otherwise circulated without the publisher's prior consent in any form of binding or cover other than that in which it is published and without a similar condition including this condition being imposed upon any subsequent purchaser.

British Library Cataloguing in Publication Data

A catalogue record for this book is available from the British Library.

ISBN 1-870332-37-7

Photoset by Inforum, Portsmouth
Printed and bound in the UK by Athenaeum Press Ltd,
Newcastle upon Tyne

Preface

Tests, assessments and intervention probes play an increasingly important role in speech and language therapy. Therapists have been helped by the provision of more critical diagnostic pointers which, in turn, help to indicate strategies for treatment and management planning. There now exists a plethora of commercially published tests with standardised scores, normative data and computerised profiles. The problem is which to choose and which to use. Practising therapists and clinicians need a test cataloguing reference book to find their way to the most useful and up-to-date information: hence the birth of *Tests of Voice, Speech and Language*.

The classification of the tests was difficult, because some tests are designed for specific client groups whereas others assess a specific disorder. Moreover, no single official classification system is accepted worldwide. It was therefore decided to list the tests in five broad categories of disorder: Voice, Articulation, Developmental disorders, Acquired disorders and Fluency.

Within each category, other tests, such as those designed for use with a related specific client group, or tests which are related in a different way to the larger category, are listed together under subheadings. Thus, for example, tests designed for use with clients with mild and severe learning disabilities, and tests assessing auditory skills in children, are listed together, under their respective subheadings, in the category Developmental disorders.

For ease of access, the tests have been organised and indexed in three ways: in the contents list at the beginning of the book the tests are listed under subheadings within the main classifications already described, alphabetically by the key word in the test's title; at the end of the book there is a title index in which all tests are listed in strict alphabetical order according to the first word of the title; and, in addition, this title index is cross-referenced to an author index, which includes second authors.

Each description of each test is organised to include the same information: age range, time taken, publisher/distributor, and aims/purpose, materials and how to administer.

In *Tests of Voice, Speech and Language*, the aim is to offer descriptions of test material which is currently available in as broad a field as possible. But not every test ever developed or published has been included. For instance, extremely expensive, rarely used, and unpublished tests have been excluded: the book is comprehensive but not exhaustive.

Because new methods and materials are constantly being developed, many tests are no longer available though in some cases revised editions have replaced the originals: in such cases the revised version is described. Moreover, changes in the publishing world have heralded changes in the distribution arrangements for some tests, particularly those from North America. Further changes are inevitable, but every effort has been made to ensure that at the time of going to press all descriptions of the materials and their availability are current. Details of the publishers are listed on pages 116–117; telephone and fax numbers have been included where appropriate, but prices have not been included as they become out-of-date so quickly. Some out-of-print tests are listed in Appendix II, together with several new tests which are in press.

Anyone wishing to supply information about new tests can photocopy page xii, fill in the details and return to the Publisher where it will be kept on file for the next edition.

I hope very much that this catalogue will prove a useful tool to all therapists, whether in clinical practice, education or research.

Myra Kersner
1992

Acknowledgements

The Test Library Catalogue of the Test Reference Library, of the National Hospital's College of Speech Sciences, London was used as the nucleus of *Tests of Voice, Speech and Language* and I wish to thank Dr Maggie Snowling, Principal of the NHCSS, for giving permission to use this material. I would also like to thank the authors who helped regarding the descriptions of many of the tests and the Librarian at the NHCSS for her help in researching the publishing details.

Contents

Preface	v
Acknowledgements	vi

Part I Voice

The Boone Voice Program for Adults	2
The Boone Voice Program for Children	2
The Buffalo III Voice Profile System	3
The Vocal Profiles Analysis Scheme	4

Part II Articulation

Screening Test for Developmental Apraxia of Speech	8
Edinburgh Articulation Test (EAT)	8
Goldman–Fristoe Test of Articulation	9
Nuffield Centre Dyspraxia Programme	10
Oral Speech Mechanism Screening Examination – Revised (OSMSE-R)	10

Part III Tests associated with developmental disorders

Cognition and symbolic understanding

Boehm Test of Basic Concepts – Revised	19
Bracken Basic Concept Scale	19
Goodenough–Harris Drawing Test	20
Raven's Progressive Matrices and Vocabulary Scales	21
Symbolic Play Test – second edition	21
Wechsler Memory Scale – Revised	22

Developmental profiles

The Schedule of Growing Skills – Developmental Screening Procedure	23
The Mossford Assessment Chart for the Physically Handicapped	24
Assessment in Nursery Education	25
PIP Developmental Charts	25
The Portage Early Education Programme	26
Pre-school Behaviour Checklist	27
Pre-speech Assessment Scale	28

Hearing and auditory

Auditory Discrimination and Attention Test	29
Wepman's Auditory Discrimination Test – second edition	30
Auditory Memory Span Test	30
Carrow Auditory–Visual Abilities Test (CAVAT)	31
Goldman–Fristoe–Woodcock Auditory Skills Test Battery – Revised edition	31
The Manchester Picture Test – Revised edition	32
Stycar Hearing Tests	33

Language

Bilingual

Sandwell Bilingual Screening Assessment	33
Sentence Comprehension Test: Revised and Panjabi editions	34

Comprehension and expression

Action Picture Test – third edition	35
Test of Adolescent Language – 2 (TOAL-2)	35
Test for Auditory Comprehension of Language – Revised edition (TACL-R)	36
Bankson Language Test – second edition (BLT-2)	36
Bristol Language Development Scales	37
British Picture Vocabulary Scale (BPVS)	38
The Bus Story – A Test of Continuous Speech – second edition	38
Carrow Elicited Language Inventory	39
Clinical Evaluation of Language Fundamentals – Revised edition (CELF-R)	40
Clinical Language Intervention Programme (CLIP)	40
Test of Early Language Development (TELD)	41
English Picture Vocabulary Test	42
Fullerton Language Test for Adolescents – Revised edition	42
Illinois Test of Psycholinguistic Abilities – Revised edition (ITPA)	43
Language Assessment Remediation and Screening Procedure (LARSP)	44
Test of Language Competence – Expanded edition (TLC – Expanded)	44
Test of Language Development – 2 Primary (TOLD-2)	45

Analysis of the Language of Learning: The Practical Test of Metalinguistics	46
Let's Talk – Inventory for Adolescents (LTIA)	46
Let's Talk – Inventory for Children (LTIC)	47
Living Language	47
Multilevel Informal Language Inventory (MILI)	48
Porch Index of Communicative Ability in Children (PICAC)	48
Pre-school Language Scale – Revised edition (PLS)	49
Receptive–Expressive Emergent Language Scale (REEL)	50
Reynell Developmental Language Scales – second revision (RDLS)	51
Reynell–Zinkin Scales for Young Visually Handicapped Children	52
South Tyneside Assessment of Syntactic Structures (STASS)	52
Stycar Language Tests	53
The Test of Syntactic Abilities (TSA)	54
Teaching Talking	55
The Token Test for Children	56
TROG – Test for Reception of Grammar – second edition	56
Test of Word Finding	57
Test of Word Finding in Discourse (TWFD)	58
Word Finding Vocabulary Scale – third edition	59

Phonology

Metaphon Resource Pack	59
PACS Pictures – Language Elicitation Materials	60
Phonological Assessment of Child Speech (PACS)	61
Phonological Process Analysis	61
South Tyneside Assessment of Phonology (STAP)	62

Pragmatics and social skills

Pragmatics Profile of Early Communication Skills	62
Test of Pragmatic Skills	63
Progress Assessment Charts of Social and Personal Development (PAC)	64
Social Skills Training with Children and Adolescents	65

Written language

The Aston Index	66
Boder Test of Reading–Spelling Patterns	66
GAP Reading Comprehension Test	67
GAPADOL Reading Comprehension Test	67
London Reading Test	67
Macmillan Individual Reading Analysis (MIRA)	68
National Adult Reading Test (NART)	69
Neale Analysis of Reading Ability – Revised British edition	69
New Macmillan Reading Analysis	70
Assessing Reading Difficulties – second edition	71
Diagnostic Spelling Test	71

Severe learning difficulties

Affective Communication Assessment (ACA)	72

Is This Autism?	73
Behaviour Assessment Battery	73
The Communication Assessment Profile for Adults with a Mental Handicap (CASP)	74
The Communication Schedule	75
The Derbyshire Language Scheme – Revised edition (DLS)	75
ENABLE – Encouraging a Natural and Better Life Experience	76
INTECOM	77
The Interactive Checklist for Augmentative Communication (INCH)	78
Personal Communication Plan (PCP)	78
Pre-feeding Skills	79
Pre-symbol Assessment	80
Pre-verbal Communication Schedule (PVCS)	80
A Clinical and Educational Manual for use with the *Uzgiris and Hunt Scales of Infant Psychological Development*	81

Vision

Carrow Auditory–Visual Abilities Test (CAVAT) see p. 31	
Developmental Test of Visual Perception – Revised edition	82
Stycar Vision Tests	82

Part IV: Tests associated with acquired disorders

Aphasia

An Aphasia Screening Test	88
The Assessment of Aphasia and Related Disorders – second edition (incorporating: The Boston Diagnostic Aphasia Examination – Revised; and The Boston Naming Test)	89
The Children's Aphasia Screening Test	90
Examining for Aphasia – Revised edition	91
Communicative Abilities in Daily Living (CADL)	91
Revised Edinburgh Functional Communication Profile (EFCP)	92
Frenchay Aphasia Screening Test (FAST)	93
The Functional Communication Profile	94
Graded Naming Test	95
Minnesota Test for Differential Diagnosis of Aphasia – Revised edition	95
Shortened Form of the Minnesota Test for Differential Diagnosis of Aphasia	96
Contributions to Neuropsychological Assessment	97
The Neurosensory Centre Comprehensive Examination for Aphasia	98
Porch Index of Communicative Ability (PICA)	99
Psycholinguistic Assessments of Language Processing in Aphasia (PALPA)	99

The Right Hemisphere Language Battery	100
The Token Test	101
Revised Token Test	102
The Western Aphasia Battery (WAB)	102

Apraxia

Apraxia Battery for Adults (ABA)	103

Degenerative disorder

Anomalous Sentences Repetition Test	104
Dysphasia/Dementia Screening Test	104
The Kendrick Cognitive Tests for the Elderly	105

Dysarthria

Frenchay Dysarthria Assessment and Computer Differential Analysis – second edition	106
Robertson Dysarthria Profile	107

Dysphagia

Dysphagia Care with Acute and Long-term Patients	107

Part V: Fluency

A Component Model	110
Assessing Communication Attitudes among Stutterers (see S24 Scale)	
Cooper Personalised Fluency Control Therapy – Revised edition	111
Assessment and Therapy Programme for Dysfluent Children	111
Systematic Fluency Training for Young Children	112
The Perceptions of Stuttering Inventory	113
S24 Scale	113
Stuttering Intervention Programme	114
Stuttering Prediction Instrument for Young Children	114
Stuttering Severity Instrument for Children and Adults	115
Appendix I: Publishers and distributors	116
Appendix II: Tests that are out of print and in press	117
Author index	119
Title index	121

If there are other tests that you would like to see included in future editions of *Tests of Voice, Speech and Language*, please photocopy, complete and send this form to Whurr Publishers Ltd, 19b Compton Terrace, London N1 2UN.

Name of Test: ....

Author: ....

Client group aimed at: ....

Publisher: ....

Year of publication: ....

Part I

Voice

The Boone Voice Program for Adults *D. Boone*	2
The Boone Voice Program for Children *D. Boone*	2
The Buffalo III Voice Profile System *D.K. Wilson*	3
The Vocal Profiles Analysis Scheme *J. Laver, S.L. Wirz and J. Mackenzie*	4

The Boone Voice Program for Adults (1982)

Author
D. Boone

Age range
Adolescents and adults

Time taken
It is not a timed assessment, and the programme is on-going

Publisher
PRO-ED, USA

Distributors
Taskmaster Ltd
Winslow Press

Aims/Purpose
The programme provides details for diagnosis and remediation of voice disorders in adolescents and adults.

Materials
The pack is in a carrying case and includes: an evaluation manual and a remediation manual; a cassette tape; voice evaluation forms; voice screening forms; voice counting charts; voice improvement recording forms; voice referral to physician sheets, and self-practice sheets. A tape-recorder will be required, but is not provided.

Administration
The programme is based on the theory and procedures outlined in Daniel Boone's book *The Voice and Voice Therapy*. The step-by-step guidelines in the remediation manual include stimulus materials considered to be age-appropriate for adolescents and adults. There are illustrated explanations of normal voice production and voice pathologies. A cassette tape contains ear training exercises. Fifteen facilitating approaches are described:
  (1) altering tongue position
  (2) change of loudness
  (3) chewing techniques
  (4) ear training
  (5) elimination of abuse–misuse
  (6) elimination of hard glottal attack
  (7) establishment of new pitch
  (8) explanation of voice problem
  (9) feedback technique
  (10) gargle effect
  (11) hierarchical analysis
  (12) open mouth technique
  (13) placing the voice
  (14) pushing exercises
  (15) yawning/sighing exercises.

The Boone Voice Program for Children (1980)

Author
D. Boone

Age range
Children from 6 to 12 years

Aims/Purpose
The programme provides details for diagnosis and remediation of voice disorders in children.

Materials
The pack is in a carrying case and comprises: a screening,

Time taken
It is not a timed assessment, and the programme is on-going

Publisher
PRO-ED, USA

Distributors
Taskmaster Ltd
Winslow Press

evaluation and referral manual which includes instructions and stimulus materials; a remediation manual; a cassette tape; voice evaluation forms; voice screening forms; voice report to parent forms; voice improvement recording forms; voice referral to physician sheets; voice tally cards; voice counting charts, and crack and peel stickers. A tape-recorder is required, but is not provided.

Administration
The programme is based on the theory and procedures outlined in Daniel Boone's book *The Voice and Voice Therapy*. The step-by-step guidelines in the remediation manual include stimulus materials and picture stickers which are of interest to children. The remediation manual includes procedures for the reduction of vocal abuse, and the search for the best voice. There are 10 facilitating approaches described:
  (1) altering tongue position
  (2) change of loudness
  (3) chewing
  (4) ear training
  (5) elimination of hard glottal attack
  (6) establishment of new pitch
  (7) open mouth technique
  (8) placing the voice
  (9) pushing exercises
  (10) yawning/sighing exercises.
The cassette is for use in conjunction with the sections on ear training and establishing new pitch.

The Buffalo III Voice Profile System (1978)

Author
D.K. Wilson

Age range
These profiles are designed to be used with children

Time taken
The profiles are not timed

Aims/Purpose
The aim of the system is to provide speech and language therapists with criteria and profiles on which to rate various parameters of voice. This information may facilitate decisions about which aspects of the child's voice may need attention, and help to establish a baseline for therapy.

Materials
The profiles, including a description, rationale and instructions for use, are written up in a book – see below.

Administration
The Buffalo III Voice Profile system consists of 10 profiles:
  (1) voice screening
  (2) group behaviour

Publisher/Distributor
The system is written up in: Wilson, D.K. (1987). *Voice Problems of Children*, 3rd edn, pp. 95–111. Baltimore: Williams & Wilkins.

(3) voice
(4) voice abuse
(5) speech anxiety
(6) resonance
(7) hearing-impaired voice
(8) voice recording
(9) voice diagnostic
(10) voice therapy progress.

There are five levels of profile criteria:
(1) normal voice
(2) mild severity
(3) moderate severity
(4) severe problem
(5) very severe.

The *Voice Screening Profile* may be used for screening large populations of children for voice problems. The *Group Behaviour Profile* allows for observation and evaluation of children in informal settings, when they may be aware/unaware that voice use is being tested. The *Voice Profile* provides a guideline for voice therapy. The *Voice Abuse Profile* lists 11 common types of voice abuse which may be rated. The *Speech Anxiety Profile* may be appraised at the same time as the voice problem. The *Resonance Profile* contains 12 items which supplement the *Voice Profile*. The *Hearing-Impaired Voice Profile* is also supplementary to the *Voice Profile* for use with all hearing-impaired people. The *Voice Recording Profile* is made at the beginning, the halfway stage and at the end of the rehabilitation programme. The *Diagnostic Profile* allows for all the relevant test and examination results to be brought forward onto one profile. The *Voice Therapy Progress Profile* enables goals and ensuing progress to be recorded.

The Vocal Profiles Analysis Scheme (VPA) (1981)

Authors
J. Laver, S.L. Wirz and J. Mackenzie

Age range
The VPA can be used with any age group and any speaker. It can be used with speakers with both normal or disordered output

Aims/Purpose
The VPA is a perceptual rating scheme for analysing long-term speaker characteristics (voice quality). Trained judges make qualitative and quantitative assessments of laryngeal and supralaryngeal 'settings' by comparing a speaker's output with specified 'neutral' settings. Neutral settings have clearly defined physiological and acoustics correlates.

Materials
Materials are only available at VPA workshops to trained judges and consist of a series of explanatory pages and a one-page protocol form on which the profile is entered.

Time taken
Untimed – about 10–15 minutes by an experienced user to complete a profile

Publisher/Distributor
The VPA is only available from tutors at workshops (see below)

Administration
A prerequisite of administration is that the user should be fully trained in the scheme. Trained users listen to a speaker (and/or tape-recording of that speaker) and rate 20 laryngeal and supralaryngeal settings in terms of the degrees of deviation from a specified neutral point. These ratings are entered on the VPA protocol form giving a graphic record of the vocal profile. Prosodic and other relevant features are also noted.

During their training, experienced listeners (speech and language therapists, voice teachers, phoneticians and others) refine their speech perceptions and analysis skills through perception by production workshops and learn:

1. About the background theory of the VPA scheme.
2. To recognise neutral settings for all parameters.
3. To rate components from the specified neutral point.

Details of distribution from: Dr Sheila Wirz/Ms Christina Shewell, National Hospital's College of Speech Sciences, London; Dr Janet Mackenzie Beck, Queen Margaret College, Edinburgh; Professor John Laver, Centre for Speech Technology, Edinburgh.

Part II

Articulation

Screening Test for Developmental Apraxia of Speech   8
R.W. Blakeley

Edinburgh Articulation Test (EAT)   8
T.T.S. Ingram, A. Anthony, D. Bogle and M.W. McIsaac

Goldman–Fristoe Test of Articulation   9
R. Goldman and M. Fristoe

Nuffield Centre Dyspraxia Programme   10

Oral Speech Mechanism Screening Examination – Revised (OSMSE-R)   10
K.O. St Louis and D.M. Ruscello

Screening Test for Developmental Apraxia of Speech (1980)

Author
R.W. Blakeley

Age range
Children from 4 to 12 years

Time taken
Approximately 10 minutes

Publisher/Distributor
PRO-ED, USA

Aims/Purpose
This test is based on an eclectic model of symptoms and may be used as a screening device to assist in differential diagnosis of apraxia of speech. It aims to indicate the need for further, more specific, speech and neurological evaluation, rather than to diagnose and label developmental apraxia.

Materials
The test consists of a manual and record forms in a sturdy box.

Administration
There are eight subtests:
(1) expressive language discrepancy
(2) vowels and diphthongs
(3) oral motor movement
(4) verbal sequencing
(5) motorically complete words
(6) articulation
(7) transpositions
(8) prosody.

These are administered to individual subjects and all scores may be marked on one record sheet. Tables are provided so that a raw score may be converted to a total weighted score. This may then be applied to a probability graph to determine whether the subject should be included in an apraxic group and thereby require further testing. Before administering any of the subtests, it is recommended that a mental age is determined, for example, from *The Peabody Picture Vocabulary Test* or equivalent, because the Apraxia Screening Test is not appropriate for subjects with severe learning difficulties.

Edinburgh Articulation Test (EAT) (1971)

Authors
T.T.S. Ingram,
A. Anthony,
D. Bogle and
M.W. McIsaac

Aims/Purpose
The EAT aims to provide '...a sensitive and economic instrument for detecting at an early age children whose command of the medium of spoken language is retarded or abnormal'. Both quantitative and qualitative assessments of articulation of consonants are possible – the latter designed to pinpoint areas in need of corrective treatment.

Age range
Children from 3 to 6 years, although it may be used with older children

Time taken
It is an untimed test, although it usually takes between 10 and 20 minutes

Publisher
Churchill Livingstone

Distributor
Longman Group UK Ltd

Materials
A soft-backed manual, record form, for both quantitative scoring and qualitative analysis, and colour picture book are provided. A tape-recorder, not provided, is essential.

Administration
Forty-one colour pictures are used as stimuli. The child is encouraged to name these spontaneously. A note is made of any responses which are imitated. All responses are recorded phonetically. Raw scores can be translated into standard scores and, if required, an articulation age. Qualitative forms are used to analyse responses under six headings, from adult form, to immature, to atypical utterance.

(A phonetic qualification, equivalent to that included in the College of Speech and Language Therapists' accredited speech and language therapy courses, is a prerequisite for users of this test.)

Goldman–Fristoe Test of Articulation (1969)

Authors
R. Goldman and M. Fristoe

Age range
Children from 2 years, to adults

Time taken
It takes approximately 30 minutes

Publisher/Distributor
NFER-Nelson

Aims/Purpose
It was designed in the USA to provide a systematic means of assessing an individual's articulation, primarily of consonant sounds. The test samples both spontaneous and imitative production and includes both single word and conversational speech production.

Materials
A manual, response forms and stimulus material, consisting of large, clear, coloured pictures, are provided in an 'Easel-kit' hard-backed ring binder.

Administration
There are three subtests:
1. *Sound-in-words* subtest, where the child produces single words in response to a stimulus picture.
2. *Sounds-in-sentences* subtest, which includes two illustrated stories to be read aloud by the examiner before the child retells the stories.
3. *Stimulability* subtest, designed in order to assess the child's ability to produce misarticulated phonemes correctly when given maximum oral and visual stimulation.

Qualitative interpretation of the results is suggested and the manual contains a section on diagnostic interpretation.

The Nuffield Centre Dyspraxia Programme (1985)

Written by:
Speech Therapy Team, Nuffield Hearing and Speech Centre

Age range
Children from 2 years. Most suitable for children from 3 to 7 years. It has been used successfully with people with mild and severe learning difficulties

Time taken
Assessment is on-going with therapy

Publisher/Distributor
The Speech Therapy Department, Nuffield Hearing and Speech Centre

For new edition, see page 118.

Aims/Purpose
The programme is aimed at children with severe speech problems when conventional/phonological therapy is not indicated. It is designed to be used by speech and language therapists, but allows for daily practice to be carried out by parents or professionals concerned with communication disorders under the guidance of the speech and language therapist.

Materials
The kit consists of a ring binder file which incorporates an assessment procedure, picture stimulus material and details of the structured programme. Instructions for administration are in a separate manual.

Administration
The child is assessed, so that an individual management programme may be planned, and in order to establish where treatment should begin. An essential part of the Dyspraxia Programme is practice for the basic oral–motor movements required for speech production. Materials are provided for constant repetition of sequences of sounds, the complexity of which is increased in small steps. Children are required to work simultaneously at different levels, in order to consolidate and stretch their sequencing abilities. Regular evaluation and reassessment is encouraged.

Oral Speech Mechanism Screening Examination – Revised (OSMSE-R) (1987)

Authors
K.O. St Louis and D.M. Ruscello

Age range
Children and adults, 5 to 70+ years

Time taken
Five to ten minutes

Aims/Purpose
OSMSE-R offers a quick and easy-to-administer screening examination of the anatomical structure and physiological functioning of the oral mechanism. It is intended to be used as a clinical instrument, although comparative data are available for both normal and deviant groups.

Materials
A manual and score sheets are provided in a box.

Administration
The assessment covers: the appearance and non-speech functions of the lips and tongue; the jaw; the teeth; the hard

Publisher
PRO-ED, USA

Distributor
Taskmaster Ltd

and soft palate; and the pharynx. The velopharyngeal mechanism, breathing and diadochokinetic rates are also examined and may be marked on the score sheets. The qualitative information gathered may be summarised and this revised edition permits separate numerical subscores for structure and function as well as a total score. Average and cut-off scores for below-average performance are provided graphically as a function of age for these scores as well as for diadochokinetic rates. Scores may be summarised and comparisons made with normative data and some clinical groups where appropriate. Recommendations may then be recorded on the sheet.

Part III

Tests associated with developmental disorders

Cognition and symbolic understanding

Boehm Test of Basic Concepts – Revised A.E. Boehm	19
Bracken Basic Concept Scale B.A. Bracken	19
Goodenough–Harris Drawing Test F.L. Goodenough and D.B. Harris	20
Raven's Progressive Matrices and Vocabulary Scales J.C. Raven	21
Symbolic Play Test M. Lowe and A. Costello	21
Wechsler Memory Scale – Revised (WMS-R) D. Wechsler	22

Developmental profiles

The Schedule of Growing Skills – Developmental Screening Procedure M. Bellman and J. Cash	23
The Mossford Assessment Chart for the Physically Handicapped J. Whitehouse	24
Assessment in Nursery Education M. Bate and M. Smith	25

PIP Developmental Charts 25
D.M. Jeffree and R. McConkey

The Portage Early Education Programme 26
R.J. Cameron and M. White

Pre-school Behaviour Checklist 27
J. McGuire and N. Richman

Pre-speech Assessment Scale 28
S. Evans Morris

Hearing and auditory

Auditory Discrimination and Attention Test 29
R. Morgan Barry

Wepman's Auditory Discrimination Test – second edition 30
J.M. Wepman and W.M. Reynolds

Auditory Memory Span Test 30
J.M. Wepman and A. Morency

Carrow Auditory–Visual Abilities Test (CAVAT) 31
E. Carrow-Woolfolk

Goldman–Fristoe–Woodcock Auditory Skills Test Battery – Revised 31
R. Goldman, M. Fristoe and R. Woodcock

The Manchester Picture Test – Revised edition 32
F.S. Hickson

Stycar Hearing Tests 33
M. Sheridan

Language

Bilingual

Sandwell Bilingual Screening Assessment 33
D. Duncan, D. Gibbs, N. Singh Noor and H. Mohammed Whittaker

Sentence Comprehension Test – Revised and Panjabi editions 34
K. Wheldall, P. Mittler, A. Hobsbaum, D. Gibbs, D. Duncan and S. Saund

Comprehension and expression

Action Picture Test – third edition 35
C.E. Renfrew

Test of Adolescent Language – 2 (TOAL-2) 35
D.D. Hammill, V.L. Brown, S. Larsen and J. Lee Wiederholt

Test for Auditory Comprehension of Language – Revised edition (TACL-R) 36
E. Carrow-Woolfolk

Bankson Language Test – second edition (BLT-2) N.W. Bankson	36
Bristol Language Development Scales M. Gutfreund, M. Harrison and G. Wells	37
British Picture Vocabulary Scale (BPVS) L.M. Dunn, L.M. Dunn, C. Whetton and D. Pintilie	38
The Bus Story – A Test of Continuous Speech – second edition C.E. Renfrew	38
Carrow Elicited Language Inventory E. Carrow-Woolfolk	39
Clinical Evaluation of Language Fundamentals – Revised edition (CELF-R) E. Semel, E.H. Wiig and W. Secord	40
Clinical Language Intervention Programme (CLIP) E. Semel and E.H. Wiig	40
Test of Early Language Development (TELD) W.H. Hresko, D.K. Reid and D.D. Hammill	41
English Picture Vocabulary Test M.A. Brimer and L.M. Dunn	42
Fullerton Language Test for Adolescents – Revised edition A.R. Thorum	42
Illinois Test of Psycholinguistic Abilities – Revised edition (ITPA) S. Kirk, J. McCarthy and W. Kirk	43
Language Assessment Remediation and Screening Procedure (LARSP) D. Crystal, P. Fletcher and M. Garman	44
Test of Language Competence – Expanded edition (TLC – Expanded) E.H. Wiig and W. Secord	44
Test of Language Development – 2 Primary (TOLD-2) D.D. Hammill and P.L. Newcomer	45
Analysis of the Language of Learning: The Practical Test of Metalinguistics E.G. Blodgett and E.B. Cooper	46
Let's Talk – Inventory for Adolescents (LTIA) E.H. Wiig	46
Let's Talk – Inventory for Children (LTIC) E.H. Wiig	47
Living Language A. Locke	47
Multilevel Informal Language Inventory (MILI) C.L. Goldsworthy	48

Porch Index of Communicative Ability in Children (PICAC)   48
B.E. Porch

Pre-school Language Scale (PLS) – Revised edition   49
I.L. Zimmerman, V.G. Steiner and R.E. Pond

Receptive–Expressive Emergent Language (REEL) Scale   50
K. Bzoch and R. League

Reynell Developmental Language Scales – second revision (RDLS)   51
J.K. Reynell

Reynell–Zinkin Scales for Young Visually Handicapped Children   52
J.K. Reynell and P. Zinkin

South Tyneside Assessment of Syntactic Structures (STASS)   52
S. Armstrong and M. Ainley

Stycar Language Tests   53
M. Sheridan

The Test of Syntactic Abilities (TSA)   54
S.P. Quigley, M.W. Steinkamp, D.J. Power and B.W. Jones

Teaching Talking   55
A. Locke and M. Beech

The Token Test for Children   56
F. DiSimoni

TROG – Test for Reception of Grammar – second edition   56
D.V.M. Bishop

Test of Word Finding   57
D.J. German

Test of Word Finding in Discourse (TWFD)   58
D.J. German

Word Finding Vocabulary Scale – third edition   59
C.E. Renfrew

Phonology

Metaphon Resource Pack   59
E. Dean, J. Howell, A. Hill and D. Waters

PACS Pictures – Language Elicitation Materials   60
P. Grunwell

Phonological Assessment of Child Speech (PACS)   61
P. Grunwell

Phonological Process Analysis   61
F.F. Weiner

South Tyneside Assessment of Phonology (STAP) S. Armstrong and M. Ainley	62

Pragmatics and social skills

Pragmatics Profile of Early Communication Skills H. Dewart and S. Summers	62
Test of Pragmatic Skills B.B. Shulman	63
Progress Assessment Charts of Social and Personal Development (PAC) H.C. Gunzburg	64
Social Skills Training with Children and Adolescents S. Spence	65

Written language

The Aston Index M. Newton and M. Thomson	66
Boder Test of Reading–Spelling Patterns E. Boder and S. Jarrico	66
GAP Reading Comprehension Test J. McLeod	67
GAPADOL Reading Comprehension Test J. McLeod and J. Anderson	67
London Reading Test	67
Macmillan Individual Reading Analysis (MIRA) D. Vincent and M. de la Mare	68
National Adult Reading Test (NART) H.E. Nelson	69
Neale Analysis of Reading Ability – Revised British edition M.D. Neale	69
New Macmillan Reading Analysis D. Vincent and M. de la Mare	70
Assessing Reading Difficulties – second edition L. Bradley	71
Diagnostic Spelling Test D. Vincent and J. Claydon	71

Severe learning difficulties

Affective Communication Assessment (ACA) J. Coupe, L. Barton, M. Barber, L. Collins, D. Levy and D. Murphy	72

Is This Autism? 73
M. Aarons and T. Gittens

Behaviour Assessment Battery 73
C. Kiernan and M. Jones

The Communication Assessment Profile for Adults with a Mental Handicap
(CASP) 74
A. van der Gaag

The Communication Schedule 75
K. Mogford

The Derbyshire Language Scheme – Revised edition (DLS) 75
W. Knowles and M. Masidlover

ENABLE – Encouraging a Natural and Better Life Experience 76
L.H. Brown and A. Keens

INTECOM 77
S. Jones

The Interactive Checklist for Augmentative Communication (INCH) 78
S.O. Bolton and S.E. Dashiell

Personal Communication Plan (PCP) 78
A. Hitchings and R. Spence

Pre-feeding Skills 79
S. Evans Morris and M. Dunn Klein

Pre-symbol Assessment 80

Pre-verbal Communication Schedule (PVCS) 80
C. Kiernan and B. Reid

A Clinical and Educational Manual for use with the Uzgiris and Hunt Scales of
Infant Psychological Development 81
C.J. Dunst

Vision

Carrow Auditory–Visual Abilities Test (CAVAT)
see p. 31

Developmental Test of Visual Perception – Revised edition 82
M. Frostig

Stycar Vision Tests 82
M. Sheridan

COGNITION AND SYMBOLIC UNDERSTANDING

Boehm Test of Basic Concepts – Revised (Boehm-R) (1986)

Author
A.E. Boehm

Age range
Children from 4 to 7 years
[*Boehm Test of Basic Concepts – Pre-school Version* covers children from 3 to 5 years]

Time taken
It takes approximately 20 to 30 minutes

Publisher
Harcourt Brace Jovanovich

Distributor
The Psychological Corporation

This replaces the *Boehm Test of Basic Concepts* (1971).

Aims/Purpose
It was designed to measure whether a child has acquired the basic concepts necessary for understanding and following the verbal directions used in a normal classroom setting, and to determine which concepts may require further instruction.

Materials
The examination kit includes a copy of each booklet and form required for testing, and directions for each, a manual, a class record, a parent–teacher conference report and a key for hand-scoring each form.

Administration
The test may be administered to a group of children or to an individual child. Two forms (C and D) cover the same 50 concepts. The child is asked to mark which of four pictures illustrates a statement given by the tester. The revised version features new norms and a new level of assessment termed 'applications' which is concerned with combinations of concepts.

Bracken Basic Concept Scale (BBCS) (1984)

Author
B.A. Bracken

Age range
Children from 2;6 to 8 years

Time taken
The Screening Test takes approximately 5–10 minutes. The Diagnostic Scale takes approximately 30 minutes

Aims/Purpose
This scale aims to identify the delayed concept development of young children and give detailed clarification of their status in relation to a wide range of concepts which are important to educational progress.

Materials
There is an examiner's manual, stimulus manual in easel format, diagnostic record forms, and a copy of screening tests A and B.

Administration
There are two elements to the scales: *The Screening Test* may be undertaken in small groups. There are 30 items on

Publisher
Harcourt Brace Jovanovich

Distributor
The Psychological Corporation

this section of the assessment. *The Diagnostic Scale* is individually administered and measures the child's grasp of 258 concepts within 10 categories:

(1) colour
(2) letter identification
(3) number
(4) shape
(5) position/direction
(6) social/emotional
(7) size
(8) texture/material
(9) quantity
(10) time/sequence.

Scoring is simple and unanimous. The Diagnostic Record Form assists analysis of each child's performance and provides a basis for the design of individualised teaching programmes.

The development of concepts identified as delayed may be aided by using the *Bracken Concept Development Programme* (1986) by B.A. Bracken, The Psychological Corporation.

Goodenough–Harris Drawing Test (1963)

Authors
F.L. Goodenough and D.B. Harris

Age range
Children from 3 to 15 years

Time taken
Approximately 15 minutes

Publisher
Harcourt Brace Jovanovich

Distributor
The Psychological Corporation

Aims/Purpose
This test aims to give a non-verbal measure of mental ability through assessment of a child's drawings.

Materials
The kit includes a test booklet, manual and quality scale cards.

Administration
The child completes a drawing of a person. This is then scored against 73 specified characteristics. Alternatively, drawings may be compared with 12 ranked drawings (Quality Scale Cards) for each of the two scales Man and Woman. The manual includes re-standardisation data for the *Goodenough Draw-a-Man Test*, the *Draw-a-Woman Scale* and an experimental *Self-drawing Scale*.

Raven's Progressive Matrices and Vocabulary Scales (1962)

Author
J.C. Raven

Age range
Children from 6 years, to adult
Standard version: 6;6–65 years
Coloured version: 6–85 years
Advanced version: 11 years to adult

Time taken
The standard version: 45 minutes
The coloured version: between 15 and 30 minutes
The advanced version: between 40 and 60 minutes

Distributors
NFER-Nelson
Oxford Psychologists Press

Aims/Purpose
The matrices aim to measure the general ability of people who may perform across a broad spectrum of ability levels, ranging from those of above-average levels to those who have little or no language, and/or mental or physical impairment.

Materials
Each package consists of a book with the relevant matrices tests, manual, appropriate vocabulary scale and record forms.

Administration
The matrices are a series of tests. There is a *standard version* for use with subjects of average abilities; a *coloured version* for use with young children, or adults with learning difficulties; and an *advanced version* for use with subjects of above-average abilities. Subjects are asked to determine which of several alternatives completes an abstract pattern; thus the subject is required to have the correct perception of shape, pattern and orientation. Each incomplete pattern and the alternatives are on a separate page in the test book, and a minimal number of verbal instructions are required.

The Mill Hill Vocabulary Scale is available for use with the standard version of the matrices. Subjects are required to define words of increasing difficulty; this provides additional information regarding their verbal ability. This scale may also provide a useful measure of pre-morbid intelligence level, for use with stroke or head-injured clients. A vocabulary scale (*The Crighton Vocabulary Scale*) is also available for the coloured version of the matrices. From the results obtained on the matrices and the scales, raw scores can be converted into percentile ranks and standardised scores which are based on normative data collated in the UK.

Symbolic Play Test – second edition (1988)

Authors
M. Lowe and
A. Costello

Aims/Purpose
To evaluate the level of representational functioning in children without using receptive or expressive language, but by examining early concept formation and the ability

Age range
Children from 1 to 3 years

Time taken
It is not a timed test but takes approximately 15 minutes

Publisher/Distributor
NFER-Nelson

to recognise and manipulate symbols in the form of miniature toys.

Materials
A small box contains a manual, record forms and a set of toys.

Administration
The toys are presented to the child in a series of four graded structured situations. As the child manipulates the toys a full record of the child's play is made on the record forms. Verbal instructions should not be required and the test should remain independent of spoken language. Scoring is objective and based on observation of what the child does with the toys. The raw scores can be translated into an age level, but the authors also advise examination of the general pattern of responses. The second edition includes a record of the results of studies with a variety of client groups which endorse the developmental play sequence on which the test is based.

Wechsler Memory Scale – Revised (WMS-R) (1988)

Author
D. Wechsler

Age range
From 16 to 74 years

Time taken
It takes approximately 45–60 minutes, including 30-minute re-test delay

Publisher
Harcourt Brace Jovanovich

Distributor
The Psychological Corporation

Aims/Purpose
This scale aims to assist in the clinical assessment of memory functioning. It may be used as a screening and diagnostic tool as part of either general neuropsychological examination, or other clinical examinations requiring assessment of memory functions.

Materials
The kit includes a manual, visual paired associates stimulus booklet, figural memory stimulus booklet, visual reproduction stimulus cards, and record forms, in a briefcase.

Administration
WMS-R has been completely revised and includes new ways of assessing and describing memory functions across the age range. *Visual memory* is tested by several new specifically designed subtests; *delayed recall* is assessed as well as short-term recall, as some subtests may be re-administered after a delay period. Five areas of *memory functions* are evaluated:

(1) general memory
(2) attention/concentration
(3) verbal memory
(4) visual memory
(5) delayed recall.

New norms in this revised version are based on a larger sampling of normal and clinical cases, stratified at nine age levels, and by gender and level of education.

DEVELOPMENTAL PROFILES

The Schedule of Growing Skills – (Developmental Screening Procedure) (1987)

Authors
M. Bellman and J. Cash

Age range
Children from 0 to 5 years

Time taken
It is not a timed procedure, but it takes approximately 20 minutes

Publisher/Distributor
NFER-Nelson

Aims/Purpose
The schedule is designed to enable health visitors, medical practitioners and clinicians to screen pre-school-aged children, and to record their developmental progress.

Materials
A lightweight carrying case contains a user's handbook and test materials required for completion of the tasks, Child Record Forms and a Profile pad. A book (by the authors above) – *The Schedule of Growing Skills in Practice* – which introduces the system, and an introductory training video are also available.

Administration
This is a comprehensive procedure, assessing development over nine skill areas. These are based on an extension of Sheridan's Stycar Sequences (see pages 33, 53, 82), thus minimal training is required. The schedule consists of the *Child Record* and the *Profile*. On the *Child Record*, 180 behaviours are listed in developmental sequence, so that only developmentally appropriate items need to be administered. The scores in each of the nine fields may be scored numerically, on these forms. The developmental screening may be repeated at intervals and the child's progress (for up to four assessments) may be marked on each form. The *Profile* provides graphic representation of these scores, giving a visual pattern of the child's development so that areas for possible intervention and remediation may be easily identified.

The Mossford Assessment Chart for the Physically Handicapped (1983)

Author
J. Whitehouse

Age range
From 5 to 18 years

Time taken
It is not a timed assessment

Publisher/Distributor
NFER-Nelson

Aims/Purpose
The chart provides a checklist of specified daily living activities which are relevant to children and young adults with mild-to-severe degrees of physical handicap. It illustrates visually their achievements and weaknesses, with particular regard to their level of independence, and may be used to aid programme planning.

Materials
The assessment comprises a soft-backed manual, record forms and transparencies of charts which may be used at case conferences.

Administration
Twelve subtests are detailed on the record charts. The areas covered are:
(1) sitting and walking
(2) mobility
(3) bathing and dressing
(4) manipulative and perceptual skills
(5) personal hygiene
(6) health
(7) communication and communication aids
(8) reading and writing
(9) mathematics
(10) financial skills
(11) domestic skills
(12) leisure and social activities.

The results of these subtests are presented in the form of a pie chart, and skills currently being learned may be indicated as well as those already mastered. Regular assessment is recommended so that comparisons of progress may be made.

Assessment in Nursery Education (1978)

Authors
M. Bate and
M. Smith

Age range
Children from 3 to 5 years

Time taken
This is an ongoing and cumulative assessment which may take place over a period of days or weeks

Publisher/Distributor
NFER-Nelson

Aims/Purpose
This assessment aims to provide nursery staff with an on-going and cumulative assessment of the development and performance skills of an individual child during the period of nursery education. The assessment reflects increasing maturation in behaviour and performance though it should not be used as a developmental guide.

Materials
The test consists of a manual, stimulus cards with black and white line drawings of pictures, figures and sequences, and shapes for copying.

Administration
Assessment is from general observation as well as from the performance of specific tasks. It may be informally administered as part of normal classroom activities. There are five main areas of assessment:
(1) social skills and social thinking
(2) talking and listening
(3) thinking and doing
(4) manual and tool skills
(5) physical skills.

Each area contains groups of assessment items which are closely related to nursery practice and may be administered to small groups of children. A small selection of items from the five areas has also been formed into four progressive stages which may be used for rapid assessment purposes. Results may be recorded on individual record sheets which are provided. The results have not been standardised. They show a description of a child's performance in the five selected areas. Progress may be checked by reassessment.

PIP Developmental Charts (1976)

Authors
D.M. Jeffree and
R. McConkey

Aims/Purpose
The aim of this assessment is that the charts should form a basis for furthering a child's development by: highlighting the developmental stage a child has just failed to reach in a particular area, and by providing a profile of development in five different areas.

Age range
Children from 0 to 5 years. Primarily designed for children with severe learning difficulties, but may be useful with other groups

Time taken
This is not a timed assessment

Publisher/Distributor
Hodder and Stoughton Educational

Materials
The charts are provided in booklet form.

Administration
The charts outline the skills which children usually develop in the first 5 years of life. The skills are grouped into five areas of development:
(1) physical
(2) social
(3) eye–hand
(4) play
(5) language.

Each area is divided into two sections. Each section starts with a target item such as 'walks confidently' beneath which are listed the skills that lead up to each item, and the approximate age at which these skills emerge. The charts are not intended for comparing a child's development with that of other children, but are designed to provide 'snapshot' assessments, and to record a child's progress over time. The booklet also includes the developmental profile.

The Portage Early Education Programme (1987)

Authors
R.J. Cameron and M. White

Age range
It has been developed specifically for use with children, age unspecified, who are developmentally delayed

Time taken
This is an on-going assessment and intervention programme

Publisher/Distributor
NFER-Nelson

[This has developed from *The Portage Project – Portage Guide to Early Education* (1976) by S. Bluma, M. Shearer, A. Frohman and H. Hilliard, but the materials are not compatible. It also incorporates the first revisions and innovations which were developed for use in the UK in *The Wessex Revised Portage Language Checklist* (1983) by M. White and K. East.]

Aims/Purpose
The Portage scheme originated in North America and was designed as a home-based programme to teach key developmental skills to children who had been diagnosed as developmentally delayed, or handicapped. It is intended that the parents carry out the programme, with planned supervision and structured support from professional workers.

Materials
There are five components to the current British edition of the Portage Programme:

1. *The Portage Early Education Programme* – a practical manual which is a ring-bound book written by R.J. Cameron and M. White.
2. *The Checklist*, including *The Portage Developmental Profile*.
3. A box of *Activity Cards*, packed in a durable case with a shoulder strap.
4. *Activity Chart* – in pads.
5. *A Parent's Guide to Early Education*, which is a book.

[Additional materials, for use in schools, which are compatible with this version of the programme, are also available from the publisher.]

Administration
1. The manual provides a basic guide to the project and the use of the materials, and serves as a basis for workshop discussions and presentations.
2. *The Checklist* is divided into six developmental areas: infant stimulation; self-help; motor; socialisation; cognitive; and language. It consists of 624 behaviours which are sequenced into years or stages of development. It facilitates the recording of existing and acquired skills. *The Portage Developmental Profile* is now included with *The Checklist*, providing a graphic representation of a child's ratings on five different areas from *The Checklist*.
3. *The Activity Cards* are colour-coded to match the developmental areas on *The Checklist*. The cards contain detailed suggestions for at least three teaching activities for each target behaviour.
4. *The Chart* has been designed by the National Portage Association to be used in conjunction with *The Checklist*. It enables more detailed task analysis and breakdown of objectives for target behaviours.
5. This book for parents also contains new UK activity cards.

Pre-school Behaviour Checklist (1987)

Authors
J. McGuire and
N. Richman

Aims/Purpose
This checklist is designed as a screening device, to provide early identification of young children with behavioural and/or emotional problems. It is for use primarily by psychologists, nursery teachers and nursery nurses.

Age range
Children from 2 to 5 years

Time taken
It takes approximately 10 minutes

Publisher/Distributor
NFER-Nelson

Materials
A see-through plastic wallet contains a slim handbook, checklists and scoring overlay.

Administration
The checklist comprises 22 items of specific behaviours which may be scored for frequency and severity. The child's scoring total is used to indicate the presence or absence of potential behavioural/emotional problems. Individual item scores provide quantified information regarding specific areas of behaviour which may be used to develop management programmes.

Pre-speech Assessment Scale (1982)

Author
S. Evans Morris

Age range
Children with neurological impairment, from birth to the normal equivalent age of 2 years, depending on the degree of handicap

Time taken
It may take 2½–3 hours to carry out a complete assessment, with a further 30 minutes being required for scoring and completing the graphs

Publisher
J.A. Preston Corporation

Distributor
Camp Ltd

Aims/Purpose
This scale has been developed to provide a method of assessing pre-speech development in neurologically impaired children. It is based on the presumption that the early development of feeding patterns, respiratory and phonatory patterns, and the movements acquired during early vocalisation, provide the foundation for the more complex act of speech production.

Materials
The scale consists of a large manual and an evaluation pack. A comprehensive list of equipment and tools which will be required is given, but no equipment is provided.

Administration
There are six components of the evaluation pack:
(1) pre-speech assessment and questionnaire for parents
(2) guiding questions for the speech assessment
(3) pre-speech assessment and summary of scores
(4) summary of scores for repeated evaluations
(5) pre-speech assessment graph
(6) pre-speech assessment scale.

The assessment considers 27 different pre-speech performance areas which have been divided into six major categories:
(1) feeding behaviour
(2) sucking
(3) swallowing
(4) biting and chewing
(5) respiration
(6) phonation and sound play.

The child's behaviour for each item is observed and recorded, and the performance is rated with a score describing the current level of ability, within the scoring range of: abnormal behaviour, normal developmental range, no behaviour. The scores may then be plotted graphically, the resulting profile indicating areas which require treatment.

HEARING AND AUDITORY

Auditory Discrimination and Attention Test (1989)

Author
R. Morgan Barry

Age range
Children from 3; 6 to 12 years (and children with moderate learning difficulties with a language comprehension age equivalent)

Time taken
It takes approximately 20 minutes

Publisher/Distributor
NFER-Nelson

Aims/Purpose
This test aims to enable speech and language therapists, language teachers and clinicians to assess a child's ability to discriminate between speech sounds. Using a minimal pairs paradigm, deficits in auditory discrimination and attention may be identified, and their potential effect on a child's speech problems may be assessed.

Materials
The test comprises a small vinyl ringbinder which opens out easel-style. There are plastic counters which may be 'posted' through holes in the binder, coloured test plates, record forms and a slim manual.

Administration
Test plates, each with two pictures (a minimal pair in terms of auditory discrimination) are presented. The words are classified according to voicing, place, manner and cluster. The child uses the counters to indicate which word of each minimal pair has been named by the tester. Each word is repeated six times in random order to check consistency of response. The numbers of trials and errors are recorded. Attention level and additional comments may also be noted on the score sheets. Using norm tables, the child's error scores may be converted into percentages and standard scores. The test was standardised on 650 children in the UK. The manual includes discussion of research studies in which the results of language-disordered children, hearing-impaired children and children with learning difficulties are compared with those of normal children.

Wepman's Auditory Discrimination Test – second edition (1987)

Authors
J.M. Wepman and W.M. Reynolds

Age range
Children from 4 to 8 years

Time taken
Although not a timed test, it takes approximately 5 minutes to administer

Publisher/Distributor
Western Psychological Services, USA

Aims/Purpose
The test aims to determine a child's ability to recognise the fine differences between the phonemes of English. It is a screening test which aims to identify children who are slow in developing auditory discriminatory skills.

Materials
The kit includes 100 test forms 1A, and 100 test forms 2A, pads and a manual.

Administration
The test items, on two alternative forms, 1A or 2A, each list 40 pairs of words. The child listens to the words and indicates verbally, or with gesture, whether the pairs consist of the same word repeated, or two different words. The alternative forms allow for re-testing. Normative data are provided based on a sample of 2000 school children in the USA. Percentile norms are given for children at half-yearly intervals from 4 to 8 years of age, and standard scores are available for each age level. The manual includes documentation regarding reliability and validity.

Auditory Memory Span Test (1973)

Authors
J.M. Wepman and A. Morency

Age range
Children from 5 to 8 years

Time taken
It is not a timed test, but only takes a few minutes to administer and score

Publisher
Western Psychological Services, USA

Aims/Purpose
This test aims to test auditory attention and recall by testing the ability to recall single syllable spoken words.

Materials
The kit comprises a manual and 200 test forms – 100 each of Form 1 and Form 2.

Administration
Single syllable nouns are presented in ordered series of two to six words for the child to repeat. The scores may then be matched with scores which have been standardised for each age group to obtain a position (between +2 and -2) on the five-point rating scale. An 'adequacy threshold' is indicated. These age related scales allow for re-testing with the same age and between ages.

Carrow Auditory–Visual Abilities Test (CAVAT) (1981)

Author
E. Carrow-Woolfolk

Age range
Children from 4 to 10 years

Time taken
The complete test takes 1½ hours to administer although subtests may be given in 5 minutes

Publisher
DLM Learning Resources, USA

Distributor
Taskmaster Ltd

Aims/Purpose
This test is designed to identify and analyse children's language and/or learning disability.

Materials
A carrying case contains three test books, copies of response/scoring booklets, an audio cassette and a manual.

Administration
There are 14 subtests which measure auditory and visual perceptual, motor and memory skills. These skills may then be analysed in-depth. Raw scores are obtained, percentile ranks and T scores. The test has been standardised on 1032 children in the USA.

Goldman–Fristoe–Woodcock Auditory Skills Test Battery – Revised edition (1976)

Authors
R. Goldman,
M. Fristoe and
R. Woodcock

Age range
From 3 to 80 years

Time taken
Approximately 15 minutes

Publisher/Distributor
NFER-Nelson

Aims/Purpose
This battery of assessment procedures aims to identify and describe auditory skills deficiencies in children and adults. It may be used in a variety of settings.

Materials
The battery comprises five hard-backed ring-bound easel kits each of which has a separate audio-cassette tape, response forms, battery profiles and manual. A portable audio-cassette recorder and earphones will be required, but are not provided.

Administration
The five kits contain the 12 tests which comprise the battery.
1. *Auditory Selective Attention Test* measures an individual's ability to attend to a task under increasingly difficult listening conditions.

2. *Diagnostic Auditory Discrimination Test Part I* measures an individual's ability to discriminate between specific sounds that are frequently confused.
3. *Diagnostic Auditory Discrimination Tests Parts II and III* are administered only to those who have shown difficulty with speech discrimination tasks in Part I.
4. *Auditory Memory Tests* consist of three separate tests which aim to measure different aspects of short-term retention and information, namely: recognition memory, memory for content and memory for sequence.
5. *Sound Symbol Tests* consist of seven tests, each designed to measure an ability which underlines the development of particular oral and written language skills.

On completion of each test, the subject's performance may be analysed in terms of percentile ranking, age-equivalent scores, standard scores and stanines. However, it must be noted that the test has been standardised on North American speakers. Furthermore, the audio-tapes are recorded by a North American speaker, and the effect this may have on the subject must be taken into account.

The Manchester Picture Test – Revised edition (1984)

Author
F.S. Hickson

[This replaces the earlier version of *The Manchester Picture Test* by T.J. Watson.]

Age range
Children from 5 years

Time taken
It is not a timed test

Publisher/Distributor
Centre for Audiology, Education of the Deaf, and Speech Pathology, University of Manchester

Aims/Purpose
It aims to assess the hearing for speech of normal hearing and partially hearing children. It is designed particularly for use with linguistically retarded children.

Materials
Picture matrices are provided and a speech trainer, or sound level indicator (not provided), is essential.

Administration
The child is asked to point to one picture out of a choice of four on each matrix. The intensity level of the stimulus word is carefully monitored. Hearing for both vowels and consonants is assessed.

Stycar Hearing Tests (1976)

Author
M. Sheridan

Age range
Children from
6 months to 8 years

Time taken
It is not a timed test but is intended to be short and fast to administer

Publisher/Distributor
NFER-Nelson

Aims/Purpose
This screening procedure is designed to obtain reliable information concerning everyday auditory competence, particularly hearing for speech, and to indicate where full diagnostic investigation is necessary. The tests included are of special value for very young children, children with severe learning difficulties, or visual difficulties, and may be used in community and school-based screening by any clinical practitioner.

Materials
A box contains the manual, test toys, coloured pictures, word sentences lists and record forms.

Administration
The comprehensive manual contains details of the procedures and materials used with different age groups. There are a series of graded hearing tests which are based on observed reactions to familiar sounds, and to everyday speech. A section of pure-tone audiometry is included.

LANGUAGE: BILINGUAL

Sandwell Bilingual Screening Assessment (1987)

Authors
D. Duncan,
D. Gibbs, N. Singh Noor and
H. Mohammed Whittaker

Age range
Children from 6 to 9 years

Time taken
Twenty minutes for each scale

Publisher/Distributor
NFER-Nelson

Aims/Purpose
This test is designed to allow non-language specialists to screen children whose first language is Panjabi and who are experiencing difficulties acquiring English as a second language. The aim of the screening assessment, which is in both languages, is to differentiate between the child who has impaired acquisition of both languages (suggesting a pathological cause) and the child who has difficulties only in acquiring English as a second language.

Materials
A plastic box with carrying handle contains the manual, picture book and presentation easel, record forms and a puppet.

Administration
Questions are asked both in Panjabi and English, concerning the 44 line drawings in the picture book. The child is required to respond verbally. The administrator must be a

fluent Panjabi speaker, but not necessarily a language specialist. A grammatical profile for each language is yielded by the error score. The total error score, when compared with the norms provided, will indicate whether the difficulty is with one or both languages. The norms provided are based on a sample of over 300 children for whom Panjabi is their first language, English their second language.

Sentence Comprehension Test: Revised and Panjabi editions (1987)

Authors
K. Wheldall,
P. Mittler and
A. Hobsbaum

Revised:
by K. Wheldall

Panjabi Edition:
D. Gibbs,
D. Duncan, S. Saund
and K. Wheldall

Age range
Children from 3 to 5 years

Time taken
It is not a timed test, but it takes approximately 15 minutes

Publisher/Distributor
NFER-Nelson

[This replaces *The Sentence Comprehension Test – Experimental Edition* (1979) by K. Wheldall, P. Mittler and A. Hobsbaum.]

Aims/Purpose
This is a picture-based screening test which aims to enable speech and language therapists and teachers to assess a child's ability to comprehend language in the absence of the contextual clues which may accompany conversation.
  The Panjabi version aims to establish whether the child's difficulties are specific to the acquisition of English as a second language, or are pathological.

Materials
There is a manual and picture book. Record forms for both the English version and the Panjabi version are provided.

Administration
The child is required to point to one of a set of pictures which most closely matches a stimulus sentence given by the assessor. Both the revised English version and the Panjabi version provide a re-standardised quantitative analysis of a child's receptive language abilities, plus a qualitative analysis of specific sentence structures which may be causing difficulties. The test correlates highly with the *British Picture Vocabulary Scale* (see page 38) and the standardised Panjabi version provides a useful comparative measure for therapists working with children for whom English is their second language. The new English standardisation is based on a sample of 300 children and the Panjabi version on 200 children for whom English is a second language.

LANGUAGE: COMPREHENSION AND EXPRESSION

Action Picture Test – third edition (1989)

Author
C.E. Renfrew

Age range
Mainly children from 3 to 7 years, although it may be used with older children

Time taken
It is not a timed test, but it takes approximately 15 minutes

Publisher/Distributor
C.E. Renfrew

Aims/Purpose
The aim of this test is to obtain short samples of spoken language which may then be evaluated in terms of the information given and the grammatical forms used.

Materials
A set of ten coloured drawings and a manual are provided. A tape-recorder may be useful, although it is not provided.

Administration
The child is asked a question relating to each picture, and the spoken response is recorded. Each response is then scored in terms of the information given, and the grammatical structures used. Scores may then be translated into age levels. Disparity between the Information and the Grammar scores, or low scores on both sections, may indicate areas for further investigation.

Test of Adolescent Language – 2 (TOAL-2) (1987)

Authors
D.D. Hammill,
V.L. Brown,
S. Larsen and
J. Lee Wiederholt

Age range
Normative data are given for students from 12 to 18;6 years

Time taken
There are no time limits, but it takes approximately 1 hour 45 minutes to administer

Publisher
PRO-ED, USA

[This is a revised version of *TOAL* 1981.]

Aims/Purpose
It aims to measure receptive and expressive language activities in adolescents.

Materials
The test comprises student books and answer booklets, summary profile sheets, and an examiner's manual.

Administration
The test assesses vocabulary (semantics) and grammar (syntax) in the areas of listening, speaking, reading and writing. The summation of scores on the subtests gives the raw scores which are then recorded onto a summary and profile sheet. This sheet also provides information about the standard scores and test scores in profile form. The scores give an adolescent language quotient based on the subtests which may be compared with other verbal cogni-

Distributor
Taskmaster Ltd

tive scores. TOAL has been standardised on students in the USA. Additional subtest items have made this revised version more appropriate for people who have language problems.

Test for Auditory Comprehension of Language: Revised edition (TACL-R) (1985)

Author
E. Carrow-Woolfolk

[This replaces the *Test for Auditory Comprehension of Language* (1973) by E. Carrow. The materials are not compatible.]

Age range
Normative data are available for children from 3 to 9 years, but TACL-R may be used with adults

Aims/Purpose
This test aims to measure auditory comprehension of language: word classes and relations, grammatical morphemes, and elaborated sentence constructions, and to determine areas of receptive linguistic difficulty.

Time taken
It takes between 10 and 20 minutes

Materials
The test comprises a 270-page test book, which includes stimulus plates each consisting of three line drawings, a 200-page manual and record forms.

Publisher
DLM Teaching Resources, USA

Administration
The child (or adult) is required to point to the drawing which corresponds to the stimulus word or sentence given by the tester. No expressive language is required of the subject. Raw scores are obtained which may be converted into standard scores, percentile ranks and age-equivalent scores. TACL-R was standardised on children in the USA.

Distributors
NFER-Nelson
Taskmaster Ltd

Bankson Language Test – second edition (BLT-2) (1990)

Author
N.W. Bankson

[This revised version replaces the *Bankson Language Screening Test*.]

Age range
Children from 3 to 6;11 years

Aims/Purpose
The new edition of this test is designed for the assessment of young children and aims to provide speech and language specialists with a measure of children's psycholinguistic skills.

Time taken
It is not a timed test

Publisher
PRO-ED, USA

Distributor
Taskmaster Ltd

Materials
The complete kit, in a cardboard box, comprises an examiner's manual, a ring-bound picture book, screen record forms and a profile/examiner's record booklet.

Administration
The test addresses three major areas: semantic knowledge; morphological/syntactical rules; pragmatics. *Semantic knowledge*: the subtests cover body parts, nouns, verbs, categories, functions, prepositions, and opposites. *Morphological/syntactical rules*: includes subtests covering pronouns; verb usage/verb tense; verb usage (auxiliary, modal, copula); plurals; comparatives/superlatives; negation; questions. Subtests in the areas of *pragmatics* cover ritualising, informing, controlling and imagining. Results may be reported as standard scores and percentile ranks, for children of the ages given above. The normative data are based on 1200 children from 19 different states in the USA. Evidence of reliability and validity is given in the manual. In addition there is a 20-item short form which is available for screening children for language problems.

Bristol Language Development Scales (1989)

Authors
M. Gutfreund,
M. Harrison and
G. Wells

Age range
Children from 15 months to 5 years who have an expressive language difficulty, including language and hearing-impaired and non-English speaking children

Time taken
This may vary, because it is not a timed assessment

Publisher/Distributor
NFER-Nelson

Aims/Purpose
The scales aim to provide a detailed analysis of children's expressive language, so that appropriate management programmes may be planned.

Materials
The set comprises a manual, main scale record forms and therapy planners.

Administration
A language sample from the child is written onto a transcription sheet. This is then analysed in terms of pragmatics, semantics and syntax so that a detailed assessment is provided of areas in which children are experiencing difficulties. Items within each section are divided into ten stages of development. The 'main scale' gives an expressive language profile, so that the user is able to assess a child's level of development at a specific age and identify areas of deficit in expressive language development. A 'syntax-free scale' is also included which has additional features that make it more appropriate for use with children who are hearing-impaired, have learning

difficulties or who are non-English speakers. The 'therapy planning form' enables the user to devise detailed intervention programmes. The scales have developed from *The Bristol Language Development Research Programme*, a longitudinal study of children from infancy to primary school as described in *Language Learning and Education* by G. Wells.

British Picture Vocabulary Scale (BPVS) (1982)

Authors
L.M. Dunn,
L.M. Dunn,
C. Whetton and
D. Pintilie

Age range
Children from 2;6 to 18 years

Time taken
It is not a timed test. Time taken will depend on which version of the test is used

Publisher/Distributor
NFER-Nelson

Aims/Purpose
The BPVS is designed to measure a subject's receptive vocabulary for standard English. It may be used in schools, for clinical work and as a research tool. It does not require the subject to read or write, and gestural responses are acceptable.

Materials
A presentation box contains the manual, the picture plates and record forms.

Administration
This test is based on the 1981 version of the *Peabody Picture Vocabulary Scales* which were standardised in North America. BPVS has been revised, updated and standardised on a UK population of English-speaking children. The child is required to point to one of four line drawings on each page, as it is named. There is a short form (38 plates) and a long form (156 plates) of this test and results of either of these are recorded on individual test records. Only items with an appropriate range of difficulty are administered. Raw scores can be converted into standardised score equivalents, percentile ranks and age equivalents.

The Bus Story – A Test of Continuous Speech – second edition (1991)

Author
C.E. Renfrew

Age range
Children from 3 to 8 years

Aims/Purpose
The test aims to assess a child's ability to produce consecutive speech. It is scored for information regarding the content, and for grammar.

Time taken
It is not a timed test

Publisher/Distributor
C.E. Renfrew

Materials
A revised manual and a booklet with the Bus Story pictures are provided. A tape-recorder is necessary, although not provided.

Administration
The tester tells the child the story, using the pictures. The child then retells the story, using the pictures as a prompt. The child's utterances are recorded, transcribed and then scored for the information given, and the sentence length. These scores may then be compared with average scores. The manual includes a section on interpretation of the scores.

Carrow Elicited Language Inventory (1974)

Author
E. Carrow-Woolfolk

Age range
Children from
3 years to 7;11 years

Time taken
It takes 30 minutes for administration and scoring. This does not include time for transcription of the tape, which has not been timed

Distributors
NFER-Nelson
Taskmaster Ltd

Aims/Purpose
This inventory aims to measure a child's production control of grammar. It is designed to enable speech and language therapists to diagnose expressive language disabilities and to identify the specific linguistic structures with which the child has difficulty.

Materials
A plastic binder contains scoring/analysis forms, verbal protocol sheets, a training guide and a manual. A training cassette is provided so that a tape-recorder is essential, though not provided.

Administration
The test is administered individually and the child is asked to imitate 52 sentences which have increasingly difficult syntactic construction. The taped responses are transcribed onto a scoring analysis form which is sectionalised to aid the error analysis of items that are substituted, added, omitted, transposed or reversed. Verbal protocol and summary sheets provide a framework for analysing the verb forms. Mean scores, percentile rankings and standard scores are given in the manual, based on data collated in the USA.

Clinical Evaluation of Language Fundamentals – Revised edition (CELF-R) (1987)

Authors
E. Semel, E.H. Wiig and W. Secord

Age range
Children from 5 to 16 years

Time taken
The full diagnostic battery takes 1 hour to complete, 30 minutes for expressive and 30 minutes for receptive language

Publisher
Harcourt Brace Jovanovich

Distributor
The Psychological Corporation

[This replaces the CELF (1980) by E. Semel and E.H. Wiig.]

Aims/Purpose
This test aims to provide a profile of the language of individual children, and to evaluate the nature and extent of language difficulties in order to facilitate the planning of remediation programmes.

Materials
A carrying case contains the examiner's manual, stimulus manual, technical manual and record forms.

Administration
There are 11 language subtests:
 (1) formulated sentences
 (2) word structure
 (3) listening to paragraphs
 (4) sentence structure
 (5) semantic relationships
 (6) sentence assembly
 (7) oral directions
 (8) word associations
 (9) word classes
 (10) recalling sentences
 (11) linguistic concepts.
The response modes are simplified for easy scoring and interpretation, and all directions, trial items and scoring guidelines are included on the record form. It has been standardised on over 2400 schoolchildren in the USA.

Clinical Language Intervention Programme (CLIP) (1982)

Authors
E. Semel and E.H. Wiig

Age range
Children from 5 to 13 years

Aims/Purpose
CLIP aims to enable professionals concerned with language development to assess over 150 defined language objectives, and to target and develop individual intervention programmes in order to strengthen areas of weakness. It provides a systematic and flexible approach to training for a comprehensive range of essential language skills.

Time taken
The assessment is not timed

Publisher
Harcourt Brace Jovanovich

Distributor
The Psychological Corporation

Materials
The complete programme includes professional's guide, a picture manual, language intervention activities manual, and progress checklists.

Administration
The programme is organised into four areas:
(1) *semantics* stresses words and word relations
(2) *syntax* emphasises word formation and sentence structure
(3) *memory* is concerned with the length and complexity of oral directions and other utterances
(4) *pragmatics* emphasises the ritualising, informing and controlling functions of language.

CLIP materials are broken down into more specific categories of form and content, and tasks are designed to elicit clearly defined intervention targets. There are full colour stimulus pictures and suggestions for the introduction and implementation of the tasks. Activities are also suggested for generalisation once the target has been achieved.

Test of Early Language Development (TELD) (1981)

Authors
W.H. Hresko, D.K. Reid and D.D. Hammill

Age range
Children from 3 to 7;11 years

Time taken
It takes approximately 15 minutes

Publisher
PRO-ED, USA

Distributor
Taskmaster Ltd

Aims/Purpose
TELD aims to measure the spoken language abilities of young children.

Materials
The complete kit includes a small examiner's manual, picture cards and record forms in a small but sturdy box.

Administration
There are 38 items on the test which assess different aspects of both receptive and expressive language. A variety of semantic tasks (testing content) and syntactic tasks (testing form) are used. On the receptive tasks the child is asked to point to specific aspects of the picture cards to indicate that they have understood both form and content. Similarly on expressive tasks, the child is asked specifically worded questions which demand specific 'form' or 'content' answers. Children are tested individually. TELD was standardised on over 1100 children in the USA. Standard scores, percentiles and age equivalents are given. Normative data are included for every 6-month interval between the ages

of 3; 0 and 7; 11 years. Validity is shown by correlation with other tests of language such as the Pre-School Language Scale (see page 49).

English Picture Vocabulary Test (1973)

Authors
M.A. Brimer and L.M. Dunn

Age range
Children from 3 to 18+ years

Time taken
It is not a timed test. It takes approximately 15 minutes to administer

Publisher/Distributor
Educational Evaluation Enterprises

Aims/Purpose
It is designed to assess the level of listening vocabulary, or the ability to recognise spoken words.

Materials
The test consists of a manual, record sheets and picture book with line drawings.

Administration
This is a British adaptation of the North American *Peabody Picture Vocabulary Scale*. The child is required to identify, by pointing, one of four pictures on a page which matches the word spoken by the tester. Raw scores can be translated into a standard score or percentile and, if required, a vocabulary age may be calculated.

Fullerton Language Test for Adolescents – Revised edition (1986)

Author
A.R. Thorum

Age range
Adolescents from 11 to 18 years

Time taken
It is not a timed test, but it takes approximately 45 minutes. It may be administered over several sessions

Aims/Purpose
This test aims to provide a quantitative and qualitative analysis of an adolescent's receptive and expressive language skills in order: (1) to distinguish between normal and language-impaired clients; (2) to indicate where the language problems may be; and (3) to suggest possible approaches to remediation.

Materials
The test comprises a slim manual, a small pack of coloured cardboard tokens, and scoring form and profile booklets.

Administration
There are eight subtests: two assess receptive linguistic processing skills: oral commands, and syllabification; six assess expressive language production skills: auditory synthesis; morphology competency; convergent production;

Publisher
Consulting Psychologists Press Inc., USA

Distributor
Oxford Psychologists Press

divergent production; grammatic competency; and idioms. The subtests need not be given in any specific order. Responses may be recorded 'plus/minus' or more descriptively. Raw scores can be compared with mean and standard deviations or with standard scores on the performance profile (standardised in the USA). The profile offers a visual record of the client's strengths and weaknesses.

Illinois Test of Psycholinguistic Abilities – Revised edition (ITPA) (1968)

Authors
S. Kirk, J. McCarthy and W. Kirk

Age range
Children from 2 to 10 years

Time taken
It is an untimed test, although it takes about 45 minutes to administer

Publisher/Distributor
NFER-Nelson

Aims/Purpose
This test aims to test children's psycholinguistic abilities; to enable the delineation of specific abilities and disabilities in young children with communication and/or learning problems, and to provide a base for the development of remedial programmes for such children.

Materials
The pack comprises all the materials necessary to administer the test, including manual, record forms and picture strips.

Administration
There are 12 subtests:
(1) auditory reception
(2) visual reception
(3) visual sequential memory
(4) auditory association
(5) auditory sequential memory
(6) visual association
(7) visual closure
(8) verbal expression
(9) grammatical closure
(10) manual expression
(11) auditory closure
(12) sound blending.

Specific instructions for administration are given for each subtest. Raw scores for each test can be translated into psycholinguistic age scores, and separate scaled scores and a profile of the child's abilities may be plotted on a graph. Normative data are based on a sample of over 1000 North American schoolchildren.
[A training course is no longer a prerequisite for use of this test.]

Language Assessment Remediation and Screening Procedure (LARSP) (1989)

Authors
D. Crystal,
P. Fletcher and
M. Garman

Age range
Adults and children

Publisher/Distributor
Whurr Publishers

Also available from bookshops

Aims/Purpose
To provide a grammatical assessment and remediation procedure which may be used with children or adults displaying various types of speech and language disabilities. The procedure is intended to provide a syntactic profile and set out stages of normal syntactic development against which abnormal development may be measured.

Materials
The LARSP procedure, introduced in 1976, is described in a paper backed book: *The Grammatical Analysis of Language Disability*, second edition (1989) by D. Crystal, P. Fletcher and M. Garman, Whurr Publishers, London.

Administration
The book outlines a descriptive syntactic model of spoken language and the development of syntax in children, as well as discussing each stage of the LARSP procedure. Profile charts (available separately*) are illustrated in the book and details are given of how to complete the charts from a transcript. Remedial sessions and case studies are also described. Use of the procedure as well as supplementary procedures is discussed in *Working with LARSP* (1979) D. Crystal, Edward Arnold, London, and *Profiling Linguistic Disability*, 2nd edition (1992) D. Crystal, Whurr Publishers, London. Several teaching procedures and sets of materials have been devised based upon the approach and it is now in use in a number of computational applications.

*Forms available from: Professor David Crystal

Test of Language Competence – Expanded edition (TLC – Expanded) (1988)

Authors
E.H. Wiig and
W. Secord

Age range
Children and adolescents from 5 to 18 years

[This replaces the *Test of Language Competence* (TLC).]

Aims/Purpose
It aims to assess metalinguistic abilities and linguistic strategy acquisition in school-aged children.

Time taken
It is not a timed test

Publisher
Harcourt Brace Jovanovich

Distributor
The Psychological Corporation

Materials
The kit includes an administration manual, a technical manual, levels 1 and 2 stimulus manuals and levels 1 and 2 record forms with portfolio.

Administration
A strategy approach to language assessment is provided by evaluating delays in the emergence of linguistic competence and in the use of semantic, syntactic and pragmatic strategies. Emphasis is placed on assessing a child's ability to perceive, interpret and respond to the contextual and situational demands of conversation in addition to basic semantic and syntactic abilities.

Test of Language Development – 2 Primary (TOLD-2) (1988)

Authors
D.D. Hammill and P.L. Newcomer

Age range
Children from 8;6 to 12;11 years

Time taken
It takes approximately 40 minutes, but it is not a timed test

Publisher
PRO-ED, USA

Distributor
Taskmaster Ltd

Aims/Purpose
This test has been designed to identify specific receptive and expressive language skills of primary school-age children. It aims to identify strengths, weaknesses and irregularities in specific areas of language development in primary age children.

Materials
The kit comprises picture plates, an examiner's manual and answer sheets.

Administration
The test covers semantics and syntax in the areas of listening and speaking. The subtests examine: sentence combining; word order; superordinate categories; and grammatic comprehension. They have sufficient reliability to be interpreted as independent entities. Raw scores are recorded and percentiles and standard scores are provided. Five quotients are generated to reflect the subject's performance relative to language constructs incorporated into the test. It has been standardised on schoolchildren in the USA.

Analysis of the Language of Learning: The Practical Test of Metalinguistics (1987)

Authors
E.G. Blodgett and
E.B. Cooper

Age range
Children from 4 to
9;11 years

Time taken
Approximately 30
minutes

Publisher/Distributor
Linguisystems Inc.,
USA

Aims/Purpose
This is a receptive and an expressive test, designed to assess the child's awareness of the structural aspects of language.

Materials
The kit includes a small examiner's manual and record forms.

Administration
There are seven tasks on the test which assess the following:
(1) ability to define concepts
(2) generating concept examples
(3) recognising concepts
(4) segmenting sentences
(5) generating words
(6) segmenting words
(7) repairing sentences.
Following the demonstration items for each task, the examiner proceeds immediately with the test items. The test is administered in its entirety to each subject, as basal and ceiling levels are not used. The examiner scores correct or incorrect responses on the response sheet provided, and uses the manual to assess age equivalents from the raw scores obtained. Percentile ranks and standard score values may be determined. The normative data were collated in the USA.

Let's Talk – Inventory for Adolescents (LTIA) (1982)

Author
E.H. Wiig

Age range
Adolescents and
pre-adolescents from
approximately 8 to
15 years

Aims/Purpose
This is designed to probe the student's ability to formulate speech acts within four communication functions: (1) ritualising; (2) informing; (3) controlling; and (4) feeling. It aims to assess communication problems and assist in the selection of appropriate teaching targets.

Materials
A picture manual, administration manual and record forms.

Time taken
These are not timed assessments

Publisher
Harcourt Brace Jovanovich

Distributor
All the items are available from The Psychological Corporation

Administration
The inventory consists of 40 items administered with a picture manual. The subject is given a brief description of the context illustrated in the picture and is then asked to suggest what the person portrayed would be likely to say. The characters portrayed are approximately 14 or 15 years of age and of multicultural origin. Forty additional items are included for those who find this task too difficult. The vocabulary of administration is at the 8-year level. Results may be linked to the intervention programmes for adolescents: *Let's Talk Intermediate Level* (1984) by E. H. Wiig and *Let's Talk – Developing Prosocial Communication Skills* (1982) by E. H. Wiig.

Let's Talk – Inventory for Children (LTIC) (1987) by E.H. Wiig is similar to the LTIA described above but is designed for use with younger children.

Living Language (1985)

Author
A. Locke

Age range
Children from pre-school age to 16 years

Time taken
Unlimited, assessment is part of the long-term teaching programme

Publisher/Distributor
NFER-Nelson

Aims/Purpose
Living Language is a remedial teaching programme designed to help children who have failed to develop spoken language skills spontaneously. It will help to identify the child's current level of language functioning and may be used by any professional to help children develop speech and language. It is particularly suited for use in small groups and may be incorporated into a school curriculum.

Materials
Booklets, manuals and appropriate recording charts for each of the three stages of the programme are provided in a hard-covered binder. An introductory video and additional picture resource materials are now also available.

Administration
The programme is divided into three stages. *Before words* is for the younger children. In this section, suggestions are provided to aid the development of pre-linguistic skills such as socioemotional development, play, listening and expressive skills. *The Pre-Language Record Booklet* is provided to record and monitor progress at this stage. *First words* is for children who are at the simple word stage but who are unable to use word combinations. A set of assessment picture cards is included and suggestions are given for assessing and expanding the child's existing vocabulary.

The Starter Programme Record Booklet is provided to record and monitor progress at this stage. *Putting words together* is intended for children who are beginning to use simple phrases and sentences. Suggestions are given for expanding the child's use of vocabulary and syntactic constructions. *The Main Programme Record Booklet* records and monitors progress of this third stage. The manual *Teaching Spoken Language* explains the principles underlying the programme which are applicable to all the stages.

Multilevel Informal Language Inventory (MILI) (1982)

Author
C.L. Goldsworthy (with probes by C.L. Goldsworthy and W. Secord)

Age range
Children from 5 to 11 years

Time taken
It is not a timed assessment

Publisher
Harcourt Brace Jovanovich

Distributor
The Psychological Corporation

Aims/Purpose
The inventory aims to identify appropriate targets for language intervention. Using informal measures of oral language, its purpose is to clarify suitable goals for language instruction.

Materials
There is an examiner's manual, picture manual and record forms.

Administration
Colourful stimulus materials are used to elicit language which is natural to the child. Three distinct levels of oral language are assessed and there are more than 50 different probes of possible intervention targets.

Porch Index of Communicative Ability in Children (PICAC) (1974)

Author
B.E. Porch

Age range
Children, unspecified age

Aims/Purpose
It is designed to quantify a child's communicative competence.

Materials
A carrying case contains: manuals, test format booklet,

Time taken
There is no limit, but it takes approximately 30–60 minutes

Publisher
Consulting Psychologists Press Inc., USA

Distributor
Oxford Psychologists Press

plastic stimulus cards, spirit masters, scoring keys, profiles and test sheets.

Administration
There is an extensive battery of tests which sample a variety of tasks representing the major input modalities – auditory and visual, – and the major output modalities: graphic, verbal and gestural. Thus inferences can be drawn about integrative ability. Scoring is based on five dimensions:
(1) accuracy
(2) responsiveness
(3) completeness
(4) promptness
(5) efficiency.
They are incorporated in 16 scoring categories. From the scores on individual items and subtests, several types of score can be computed such as overall response level, mean scores for subtests, and general communication level.

(In order to gain maximum benefit from use, clinicians are urged to attend training workshops, or to obtain training from an experienced user. Information regarding training from: PICA Workshops.)

Pre-school Language Scale – Revised edition (PLS) (1979)

Authors
I.L. Zimmerman, V.G. Steiner and R.E. Pond

Age range
Children from 1 to 7 years. It may also be used with older children who are assumed to be functioning at a pre-school or primary language level

Time taken
It takes approximately 20 minutes

Aims/Purpose
The PLS is an evaluation and screening instrument which may be used to diagnose and isolate the strengths and deficiencies of a child's auditory and verbal language. It may be useful in helping to develop language programmes and to select individual children for speech and language therapy.

Materials
The test materials comprise a PLS manual, a colourful picture book and record forms. Specific named items required for testing are not supplied.

Administration
The test assesses both *auditory comprehension* (AC) and *verbal ability* (VA) and consists of a series of auditory and verbal tasks, each of which is assigned to a certain age level. The tasks measure: discrimination, grammar and vocabu-

Publisher
Harcourt Brace Jovanovich

Distributor
The Psychological Corporation

lary, memory and attention span, temporal/spatial relations and self-image, in both domains. The AC tasks determine whether the child can receive auditory information and indicate this reception by a meaningful non-verbal response. The VA items measure a child's responses to a series of graded tasks. This section includes specific items designed to test articulation. AC age and VA age can be calculated and converted to quotients which represent the ratio of these ages to the chronological age. Language age may also be computed. The PLS profile and checklist included in the score sheet summarise the child's performance and illustrate the child's language status on the PLS. The age levels obtained represent the point at which most children have achieved such competency and are not directly comparable to mental ages established on psychological tests of intelligence. Validity and reliability studies were carried out on 5230 children in the USA.

Receptive–Expressive Emergent Language Scale (REEL Scale) (1971)

Authors
K. Bzoch and R. League

Age range
Children from 0 to 3 years

Time taken
It is an untimed test, although may take approximately 10 minutes

Distributors
NFER-Nelson
Winslow Press

Aims/Purpose
The test aims to determine whether expressive and receptive language skills are following normal developmental patterns during the first 36 months of life. It may aid speech and language therapists to screen young children and prioritise waiting lists.

Materials
A handbook and record forms are provided.

Administration
The test consists of an outline of developmental stages for receptive and expressive language presented in 22 sections. There are three receptive and three expressive items per section and these are divided across the age bands so that twelve items apply to year 1, six apply to year 2 and four apply to year 3. The tester obtains the information required to complete the form from an interview with a parent or carer, as well as from observation of the child. Language ages, or quotients, are obtained for receptive or expressive language individually, or as a combined overall language age/quotient. The manual includes theoretical discussion and guidelines for interpretation of the results.

Reynell Developmental Language Scales – second revision (RDLS) (1985)

Author
J.K. Reynell

Revised edition:
M. Huntley

Age range
Children from 1 to 7 years

Time taken
Although it is not a timed test, it takes approximately 30 minutes

Publisher/Distributor
NFER-Nelson

Aims/Purpose
RDLS aims to assess, as independently as possible, expressive language (EL) and verbal comprehension (VC 'A' and VC 'B') during the years that are most important for language development. The VC 'B' scale allows for the assessment of verbal comprehension in severely physically handicapped or withdrawn children.

Materials
A strong carrying case contains a comprehensive manual, record forms for both VC and EL and a set of toys and pictures.
(A conversion kit containing the revised manual and picture cards is available, which may be used with the toys and objects of the earlier version of the RDLS.)

Administration
The battery comprises three scales. On the VC 'A' scale the child is asked to point to or manipulate toys in response to commands of increasing length and/or complexity. There are ten sections arranged in developmental order which assess understanding from single words to complex instructions. For children unable to use their hands, VC 'B' allows for eye pointing responses. On the EL scale 25 activities are arranged in three sections each concerned with a different aspect of language. The sections are arranged in the developmental order: pre-symbolic stage; naming and ability to describe word meanings; the use of language to express consecutive ideas. These stages may overlap. For assessment EL, naming and description of objects and pictures, and explanation of spoken words are required. Observation and recording of the child's spontaneous expression during the assessment are recommended. The scales provide a qualitative as well as quantitative measure. Raw scores can be converted into standard scores or age-equivalent scores. The test has been standardised in the UK on a sample of over 1300 children between the ages of 18 months and 7 years.

[Speech and language therapists are required to complete a training course before using the materials.]

Reynell–Zinkin Scales for Young Visually Handicapped Children (1979)

Authors
J.K. Reynell and
P. Zinkin

Age range
Visually handicapped children from birth to 5 years, who may or may not have additional handicaps

Time taken
It is not a timed test, but takes approximately 20 minutes

Publisher/Distributor
NFER-Nelson

Aims/Purpose
These scales are intended to give guidelines for assessment and developmental advice. They aim to assess the child's level in terms of intellectual processes established rather than skills acquired, and explore the areas of learning and development which are considered particularly important for visually handicapped children so that an individual programme of help may be planned.

Materials
The test consists of a small soft-backed manual and record forms. A list and photographs of items which may be suitable as test materials are given in the manual, but it is essential that the test remain flexible and choice of the items is left to the individual examiner according to the relevance of each child's needs.

Administration
Explicit directions for administration are given in the manual for each subscale, and criteria are given for scoring the record sheets. Several aspects of intellectual development are assessed through the subscales:
(1) social adaptation
(2) sensory–motor understanding
(3) exploration of environment
(4) response to sound and verbal comprehension
(5) vocalisation and expressive language
(6) vocabulary and content
(7) communication
(8) expressive communication.

A profile may be gained from the overall assessment from the subscales. An equivalent age may be computed from the raw score totals but standardisation is difficult owing to the nature of the test and no reliability studies have been attempted.

South Tyneside Assessment of Syntactic Structures (STASS) (1988)

Authors
S. Armstrong and
M. Ainley

Aims/Purpose
STASS is a rapid assessment procedure used to elicit and highlight potential areas of difficulty within a child's expressive language. It examines the range of grammatical

Age range
Children from 3 to 7 years

Time taken
Approximately 12–15 minutes

Publisher
STASS Publications

Distributors
STASS Publications
Winslow Press

structures produced by a child, but only in the context of the assessment.

Materials
The assessment comprises a small book containing laminated pages of pictures. The prompt questions for each of the pictures is on the back. The book also contains all information needed to carry out the procedure. There are photocopiable assessment forms. A tape-recorder is required, but not provided.

Administration
The 32 coloured pictures are presented to the child with one or two prompt questions. These should be asked exactly as written, but may be repeated as often as necessary. The child's responses are recorded verbatim on the data forms, and a tape-recording of the assessment is essential to check the accuracy of the transcribed data. The assessment has been designed to elicit structures at clause, phrase and word level in stages I to IV of LARSP (see page 44). Profiles of the structures produced by normal 3-, 4- and 5-year old children are provided for comparison, and the data elicited can be analysed in two ways. Using the rapid scoring technique, it may be quickly scanned for the presence/absence of grammatical structures. This will provide a quick screening assessment. Alternatively, a Detailed Analysis Form may be used to give a more comprehensive picture of the child's use of language. The authors point out that whilst the child *can* produce, it does not make any statement about those structures that are absent from the data sample.

Stycar Language Tests (1976)

Author
M. Sheridan

Age range
Children from 1 to 7 years

Aims/Purpose
This screening test has been devised for use by paediatricians and professionals interested in communication, to help in the differential diagnosis of young children with speech disorders, or older children with learning difficulties. The test aims to provide information regarding reception, comprehension and expression, of spoken language and other forms of communication.

Time taken
It is not a timed test, but will take approximately 30 minutes

Publisher/Distributor
NFER-Nelson

Materials
A large box contains the manual, common objects, miniature toys and a picture card booklet.

Administration
The test consists of three overlapping procedures. *The Common Objects Test* assesses the child's ability to name and describe objects, relate them together and demonstrate an understanding of their use. *The Miniature Toys Test* assesses understanding and creativity in the use of language codes. *The Picture Book Test* provides information about many aspects of communication including verbal reception, auditory discrimination, auditory memory, sound sequencing, articulation, vocabulary, imitation of speech sounds, speech sequencing, words and narrative, grammar and syntax. The test is not designed to produce a numerical quotient and considerable clinical experience may be necessary in order to interpret the findings.

The Test of Syntactic Abilities (TSA) (1978)

Authors
S.P. Quigley,
M.W. Steinkamp,
D.J. Power and
B.W. Jones

Age range
Prelingually, profoundly deaf students from 10 to 19 years of age, although it may also be used for people with various types of learning disabilities who have a reading level of approximately 2.0

Aims/Purpose
The TSA was designed as a diagnostic tool for therapists and educators working with linguistically impaired deaf children, although it may also be appropriate for assessing children with linguistic difficulties, and for those for whom English is a second language. TSA assesses children's difficulties in comprehending and using the syntactic structures of standard English. It may also be used as an aid when planning a remediation programme.

Materials
A large box contains index cards of assessment materials. There is a slim soft-backed manual.

Administration
TSA consists of: a diagnostic battery of 20 individual tests, each of which contains 70 multiple choice items; and a screening test containing 120 items selected from the diagnostic battery. The 20 diagnostic tests cover 9 major syntactic structures of English:
(1) negation
(2) conjunction
(3) determiners
(4) question formation
(5) verb processes

Time taken
The diagnostic battery takes approximately 30 minutes per test. This will need to be completed over several sessions. The screening test may take approximately 1 hour

Publisher/Distributor
PRO-ED, USA

(6) pronominalisation
(7) relativisation
(8) complementation
(9) nominalisation.

Each test includes groups of items which examine the stages of development of the syntactic structure covered. The screening test provides a profile of a child's strengths and weaknesses on the syntactic structures and their component forms. The information may then indicate which structures need to be examined in depth and thus may be used as a guide when planning remediation. Raw scores are converted to percentile ranks and age equivalents. The test was standardised in the USA and normative data are given for prelingually, profoundly deaf students from 10 to 19 years of age.

Teaching Talking – A Screening and Intervention Programme for Children with Speech and Language Difficulties (1991)

Authors
A. Locke and M. Beech

Age range
Children from 3 to 11 years

Time taken
The assessment is not timed and the intervention programme is on-going

Publisher/Distributor
NFER-Nelson

Aims/Purpose
This programme is designed for speech and language therapists, teachers and educational psychologists, working in nurseries or mainstream schools. It enables them to identify children who are experiencing difficulties with communication, and provides a structured programme for intervention in the classroom.

Materials
A plastic wallet contains: a teaching procedures handbook, which includes photocopy masters of all screening materials; a teaching resources handbook, and record forms and profiles for nursery, infant, and junior school-aged children.

Administration
The teaching procedures handbook outlines the philosophy and development of teaching talking. Three stages are described:
(1) initial screening
(2) assessment of language skills and initial intervention
(3) detailed assessment and intervention.
The initial screening encourages the use of observation of the child in the classroom setting, in order to identify children with communication difficulties. The language support skills profiles then enable the teacher/therapist to further assess language skills and plan small group interven-

tion programmes for these children. There is a more detailed assessment and intervention programme for children who continue to experience difficulties which may also be used to monitor and evaluate progress. Various abilities related to language skills may be plotted on the record forms according to given criteria. These include: play and social development; listening and understanding; pre-language; emerging language; and interaction. Results may then be brought forward onto the quick indicator and detailed profiles. The teaching resources handbook contains activities which may be included in the programme.

The Token Test for Children (1978)

Author
F. DiSimoni

Age range
Children from 3 to 12 years

Time taken
It takes approximately 30 minutes

Publisher
DLM Teaching Resources, USA

Distributors
NFER-Nelson
Taskmaster Ltd

Aims/Purpose
The test was developed in order to find 'more adequate data for the performance of children' on an adaptation of the De Renzi and Vignolo's *Token Test* as described for use with adults (see page 101). It aims to try to identify the presence of receptive language dysfunction in children.

Materials
The test is in a box containing small tokens of differing colours and shapes, record forms and a slim manual.

Administration
The Token Test is divided into subtests, involving commands for moving the tokens. These commands become progressively more complex and later subtests need not be administered if numerous errors are scored on Part 1. Age and grade norms (standardised in the USA) indicate the presence and possible severity of a receptive language deficit. It is recommended that a child thus identified is referred for more detailed assessment.

TROG – Test for Reception of Grammar – second edition (1989)

Author
D.V.M. Bishop

Aims/Purpose
This test is designed to assess children's understanding of grammatical contrasts in English and to compare their comprehension of individual structures with that of their peers. It may be useful in the assessment of children with speech and language disorders, deafness, severe/moderate

Age range
Normative data are available for children from 4 to 12 years. Some normative data for adults are also available

Time taken
Ten to 20 minutes

Publisher/Distributor
Dr D. Bishop, University of Manchester

learning difficulties and cerebral palsy, as well as in the assessment of adults with acquired dysphasia. It aims to pinpoint areas of specific difficulty and to provide a profile of patterns of errors.

Materials
There is a soft-backed picture manual, manual and score sheets. Vocabulary picture cards are also provided.

Administration
The vocabulary cards may be used as a pre-test to ensure the subject's familiarity with the vocabulary. Each set of four line drawings on each page of the picture book tests the understanding of a specific type of grammatical contrast. The contrasts are arranged in increasing order of difficulty. The subject chooses one of the four pictures which corresponds to a phrase or sentence spoken by the tester. No expressive language is required from the subject. Results may be interpreted as centile scores which allow statistical comparison of each child's performance with normal children of the same age. Raw scores may be converted to standardised scores and age-equivalent scores may be obtained if required. The test has been standardised on over 2000 British children aged 4 to 12 years. Some adult norms are also given.

Test of Word Finding (1986)

Author
D.J. German

Age range
Children from 6;6 to 12;11 years. This includes children who have learning difficulties or language disorders

Time taken
Approximately 20–30 minutes

Aim/Purpose
This test has been designed to assess children's word-finding skills and to determine whether a child's expressive language problem is a result of word-retrieval difficulties. It aims to help in remediation planning and evaluation of progress.

Materials
The kit comprises an easel-binder test book containing coloured graphics, administration, interpretation and scoring manual, and technical manual, response booklets. If the Actual Item Response Times are to be measured, an audio cassette recorder and stopwatch will be required.

Administration
The child is presented with naming tasks from a test book of pictures so that his or her accuracy and speed in naming may be measured. Procedures are included for analysing the nature of the naming response and describing the naming

Publisher
DLM Teaching Resources, USA

Distributor
Taskmaster Ltd

behaviour, including observing the presence of secondary characteristics such as gestures and extra verbalisation. There are six sections tested:
(1) picture naming: nouns
(2) sentence completion naming
(3) description naming
(4) picture naming: verbs
(5) picture naming: categories
(6) comprehension assessment.

Responses are recorded in individual booklets. An accuracy score summary gives total raw scores which may then be converted to standard scores and percentile ranks. Results may be compared with normative data researched in the USA. The word-finding profile may be completed by plotting the child's Estimated/Actual Item Response Time.

Test of Word Finding in Discourse (TWFD) (1991)

Author
D.J. German

Age range
Children from 6;6 to 12;11 years

Time taken
Approximately 15–20 minutes

Publisher
DLM Learning Resources, USA

Distributor
Taskmaster Ltd

Aims/Purpose
This test has been designed as a diagnostic test to assess word-finding skills in discourse.

Materials
The complete test comprises an examiner's manual which includes stimulus pictures, and test record forms. A tape-recorder is required but is not provided.

Administration
There are three stimulus pictures which may be used together with standard auditory prompts to encourage the child to tell a story. The child's language during this story telling may be recorded and transcribed. The test includes a model for analysing the child's word-finding skills as demonstrated during the narrative. The procedure has been standardised on 856 subjects in the USA, so that the child's narrative may be compared with normative data. A non-standardised procedure may also be used with children outside the age range for which normative data are available. This follows the same format, but may include other visual stimuli. The scores give a Productivity Index, which measures quantitatively how much language is produced; a Word-Finding Behaviours Index – which measures the frequency of specific word-finding behaviours such as repetitions, reformulations, substitution and insertions. Percentile ranks and Standard Scores may be obtained for both of these indices.

Word Finding Vocabulary Scale – third edition (1988)

Author
C.E. Renfrew

Age range
Children from 3 to 8 years

Time taken
It is not a timed test, but it takes approximately 10 minutes, as there is usually a definite cut-off in correct responses

Publisher/Distributor
C.E. Renfrew

Aims/Purpose
This test aims to assess the child's ability to use nouns to name pictures. It is not intended to test phonology and has been devised so that it may be used with children with severe speech difficulties. The pictures are arranged in order of difficulty as found by the frequency of correct response.

Materials
The test consists of a set of 45 line drawings on cards, scoring sheets and a manual.

Administration
The child is asked to name the object on each card and the response is recorded. Raw scores may then be translated into age levels.

LANGUAGE: PHONOLOGY

Metaphon Resource Pack (1990)

Authors
E. Dean, J. Howell, A. Hill and D. Waters

Age range
Children from 3;6 to 7 years

Time taken
Screening: administration and analysis take approximately 20 minutes
Monitoring: administration and scoring time is approximately 5 minutes

Publisher/Distributor
NFER-Nelson

Aims/Purpose
This is a comprehensive assessment and treatment approach for children with phonological disorders. The assessment uses phonological process analysis procedures. The treatment procedure is based on linguistic and learning theory, and aims to bring about phonological change through development of metalinguistic awareness, i.e. the children's knowledge of language.

Materials
The Metaphon Resource Pack contains a manual, a screening picture book, screening record forms, probe picture book, probe record booklets and a set of monitoring pictures, in a carrying case.

Administration
There are three distinct parts to the assessment procedure. All three parts use a picture naming format.
1. *Screening*: this provides a quickly administered overview of any problems a child may be encountering in phonological development.

2. *Probing*: specific probes enable a very detailed assessment to be made of any potential problems identified during the screening procedure.
3. *Monitoring*: this very quickly administered procedure can be repeated at regular intervals during a period of treatment to monitor the extent and nature of phonological change.

The results of the assessment provide quantitative and qualitative information to determine and monitor the focus of treatment.

PACS Pictures – Language Elicitation Materials (1987)

Author
P. Grunwell (with Grimsby Health Authority, Department of Speech Therapy)

Age range
Children of any age

Time taken
Approximately 20 minutes; at least two sessions may be required

Publisher/Distributor
NFER-Nelson

Aims/Purpose
PACS pictures have been specifically designed so that the whole range of the target adult phonetic system is represented. The aim of using the materials is to elicit a spontaneous and representative speech sample of the child's habitual speech patterns which may be used for screening/assessment purposes.

Materials
The pack comprises a manual, record booklets and a picture book in a ring binder.

Administration
The pictures are designed to interest children across sociocultural boundaries. They alternate between composite and thematic (e.g. semantic) collections. Forty-one words from the Edinburgh Articulation Test (see page 8) have been included in the materials. The speech sample produced by the child when describing the picture may be used as a quick screening device, or it may be helpful in more detailed linguistic analyses and assessments such as PACS (see page 61). Details regarding the application of PACS analysis to the 200 word list are provided in the manual. It is advisable to take 'live' transcriptions as well as audiotapes. The manual includes guidelines and suggestions for how to use the material successfully.

Phonological Assessment of Child Speech (PACS) (1985)

Author
P. Grunwell

Age range
Children (no age specified)

Time taken
This may vary according to the method of analysis used

Publisher/Distributor
NFER-Nelson

Aims/Purpose
PACS aims to provide a detailed phonological analysis of children's speech which will aid diagnosis and treatment planning.

Materials
The kit comprises a manual and photocopy masters of analysis worksheets in a plastic folder.

Administration
The manual offers guidelines regarding how to obtain and record a representative speech sample. Two different approaches are suggested for analysis of the data, according to the sample taken. Comparisons may be made of the child's sound system with that of an adult, and with the sound system 'normally' expected in children at the same developmental stage. The data interpretation is organised to give diagnostic indications and to provide a framework for planning a remediation programme. Samples, worked examples and exercises are given to allow for practice in the procedure. The two main approaches are contrastive analysis and phonological process analysis. In addition, work sheets are provided for the analysis of communicative adequacy, polysystemic phonotactic analysis and for phonetic analysis.

Phonological Process Analysis (1979)

Author
F.F. Weiner

Age range
Children from 2 to 5 years

Time taken
It is untimed, but may continue for more than one session

Publisher/Distributor
PRO-ED, USA

Aims/Purpose
This is intended to be used as a diagnostic tool for children with communication problems. It aims to provide a profile of the child's phonological system, by stimulating English speech sounds in a variety of phonetic contexts.

Materials
The manual includes 136 cartoon-like action pictures with instructions for their use in stimulating speech. A sample scoring sheet and process profile are also included – further sheets and profiles are available separately.

Administration
Results present a pattern of phonological processes and there is a detailed chapter of how to interpret the profile and consider remediation, on the basis of the analysis.

South Tyneside Assessment of Phonology (STAP) (1988)

Authors
S. Armstrong and M. Ainley

Age range
Unspecified

Time taken
Approximately 15 minutes

Publisher
STASS Publications

Distributors
STASS Publications
Winslow Press

Aims/Purpose
This is a rapid screening assessment used to obtain a profile of a child's phonological system. The material aims to elicit consonant phonemes and consonant clusters within the contexts of word initial, medial (i.e. all intervocalic) and final positions.

Materials
A small laminated book contains 27 coloured pictures of objects. There are brief instructions for using and scoring the assessment. Photocopiable recording forms and analysis forms are also included.

Administration
The child is required to name the items as presented; where the picture contains a number of objects within a contextual setting, the assessor points to each item. The target words are listed on the recording forms, and the child's responses are recorded and transcribed, using phonetic transcription with diacritics as necessary. Two analysis forms are provided for easy identification of problem phonological areas; one is for single consonants and one for clusters. The second form provides space for recording the different contexts in which a phoneme occurs.

LANGUAGE: PRAGMATICS AND SOCIAL SKILLS

Pragmatics Profile of Early Communication Skills (1988)

Authors
H. Dewart and S. Summers

Aims/Purpose
The Profile aims to provide a descriptive, qualitative assessment of the pragmatic aspects of language. It may be used by any professional who has an interest in the development of language and communication, and will help in treatment planning where pragmatics need to be part of the therapy programme.

Materials
It is a soft-backed spirally bound book which includes photocopy master sheets of the structured interview.

Age range
Children from 9 months to 5 years. It may be appropriate for bilingual, hearing-impaired, non-verbal and/or physically handicapped children, as well as for children with severe learning difficulties

Time taken
Thirty minutes, but it may be administered over several sessions

Publisher/Distributor
NFER-Nelson

Administration
The Profile affords a qualitative overview of: how children express their communicative intent; how they respond to communication; and how they participate in conversation in a wide range of communicative settings. It evaluates the impact of situational contexts on children's communication. It offers insight and information regarding intervention and can be used to evaluate the success of therapy in this area. Each individual profile is achieved through a structured though informal interview with the parent/carer. The interview covers four main areas:
1. *Communicative Intentions*, which covers both range and form.
2. *Response to Communication*, which includes the type of input responded to as well as the nature of the response.
3. *Interaction and Conversation*, which looks at the extent, form and effectiveness of the child's contribution.
4. *Contextual Variation*, such as time, topic, place and partner.

The resultant profile offers insight regarding the child's communication outside the classroom or clinical setting.

Test of Pragmatic Skills (1985)

Author
B.B. Shulman

Age range
Children from 3 to 8 years

Time taken
It is not a timed assessment

Publisher/Distributor
Communication Skill Builders, USA

Aims/Purpose
The test was designed for use with children whose use of conversational intentions is limited, or is impaired. It aims to provide a standardised/norm-referenced assessment measuring a specific set of conversational behaviours– conversational intentions.

Materials
The test consists of a manual and relevant score sheet booklets. Audio (or video) facilities may be useful if available.

Administration
The test focuses on 10 conversational intentions:
(1) requesting information
(2) requesting action
(3) refusing and denying
(4) naming/labelling
(5) answering/responding
(6) informing
(7) reasoning

(8) summoning/calling
(9) greeting
(10) closing conversation.

The tester observes the child's performance as listener, and the child's performance as speaker on four standardised tasks. The tasks centre round playing with puppets; copying line drawings with pencil and paper; playing with telephones; and building models with blocks. Specific probes are introduced to try to elicit from the child illocutionary acts such as: greeting; naming; answering; or informing. Sample responses are given. The child's responses are recorded and scored on a rating scale of 0 ('no response') to 5 ('contextually appropriate response with extensive elaboration'). A raw score of total ratings from the probes may be computed to produce a mean composite score for the four tasks. This may then be used to determine a percentile ranking for the child's performance. The test was standardised on a sample of 650 children in the USA aged 3 to 8;11 years. A *Language Sampling Supplement* is an optional addition, suggesting ways in which to examine verbal turn-taking, speaker dominance, topic maintenance, and topic change. Thus the tester may gather further information regarding the child's conversational abilities.

Progress Assessment Charts of Social and Personal Development (P-A-C) (1963)

Author
H.C. Gunzburg

Age range
For people of all ages who have learning difficulties

Time
It is not a timed assessment

Publisher
SEFA (Publications) Ltd

Distributor
MENCAP Bookshop

Aims/Purpose
These charts are designed to describe qualitatively the strengths and weaknesses of an individual with learning difficulties in relation to others with similar difficulties, over four areas of social competence. The purpose is that the information provided will allow appropriate remedial action to be planned.

Materials
The materials consist of a soft-backed manual and charts.

Administration
Charts are available for three levels:
1. Primary PAC for young children.
2. PAC Form I for older children.
3. PAC Form II for adolescents and adults.

Each chart, presented in a circle diagram form, is an inventory of 120 skills. These skills are divided into four areas: self-help; communication; socialisation; and occupation.

The skills are graded according to difficulty from the centre of the circle to the periphery. Spaces in the diagram referring to the specific skills achieved by an individual are shaded by the examiner and thus a clear picture of social competence can be achieved. In addition, more recent editions of the charts indicate either progressive learning, or competence in the application of complex living skills. On completion of the chart, appropriate training and educational programmes may be designed in order to improve social and personal functioning.

Social Skills Training with Children and Adolescents (1980)

Author
S. Spence

Age range
Children and adolescents from 5 to 16 years

Time taken
It is not a timed assessment

Publisher/Distributor
NFER-Nelson

Aims/Purpose
The manual aims to provide the basis for a structured programme of social skills training.

Materials
The package consists of a soft-backed manual, a set of photo cards related to specifically identified social skills, and appropriate record forms.

Administration
Different methods of assessing social skills are discussed in the manual: Staff Questionnaire; Self-report Questionnaire; Direct Behaviour Questionnaire; and the Assessment of Emotional Perception. Photo cards are used for assessing the perception of emotion. The manual also includes techniques for teaching social responses and gives outlined examples of activities, games and role-play which may be used in the assessment of social skills. There are five record forms on which students' responses may be recorded:
(1) perception of emotion from facial expression
(2) perception of emotional expression from voice quality cues
(3) list of social situation problems
(4) social behaviour at school
(5) staff questionnaire of social behaviour.
The data can then be summarised on an assessment chart so that an individual's key skill areas of strengths and need may be readily identified.

LANGUAGE: WRITTEN

The Aston Index (1976)

Authors
M. Newton and
M. Thomson

Age range
Children from 5;6 to 14 years, although it can be used with older children and young adults

Time taken
Between 30 and 45 minutes

Publisher/Distributor
LDA

Aims/Purpose
The Index aims: 'to provide a profile of the child's ability to cope with the vital skills that written language requires'. It may be used on two levels: Level I, as a screening procedure to enable early diagnosis of potential reading/writing problems by examining pre-reading skills; Level II as a diagnostic procedure for children over 7 years who are not making expected progress in reading, spelling and writing.

Materials
A large cardboard box contains a manual, test cards, most of the test materials required, instructions and scoring forms.

Administration
For each of the 16 tests there is a test card which indicates clearly the objective of the test, the materials required, and instructions regarding administration and scoring. The tests covered include: visual sequential memory; sound blending; discrimination; vocabulary; reading and spelling. The results of the tests can be plotted graphically.

Boder Test of Reading–Spelling Patterns (1982)

Authors
E. Boder and
S. Jarrico

Age range
Children from 6 years, to adults

Time taken
It is not timed, but takes approximately 30 minutes

Publisher
Harcourt Brace Jovanovich

Aims/Purpose
This test was designed to be used as a diagnostic screening device to identify normal/abnormal reading and spelling patterns. It enables the abnormal patterns to be classified into subtypes, thus providing pointers for remediation.

Materials
A box contains the spirally bound manual, students' forms and record forms for the reading test; test forms and sentences to be dictated for the spelling test; alphabet tasks record forms; and diagnostic summary forms.

Administration
A systematic sequence of reading/spelling tasks of word lists and sentences is given, in order to identify four subtypes of reading disability. The test results are both qualitative and

Distributor
The Psychological Corporation

normative, offering a systematic way of comparing the reading and spelling patterns of the student with those of normal readers. They also differentiate specific reading difficulties from reading difficulties which may be due to physical, mental, emotional or educational impairment.

GAP Reading Comprehension Test (1983)

Author
J. McLeod

Manual:
by D. Unwin

Age range
Children from 7;8 to 12;6 years

Time taken
Approximately 30 minutes, depending on the age of the child

Publisher/Distributor
Heinemann Educational

Aims/Purpose
GAP aims to assess a child's reading comprehension through the cloze technique.

Materials
The kit includes a scoring manual and forms B and R which are parallel tests.

Administration
The child is required to replace, correctly, words which have been deleted at random from seven passages. The passages are graded in difficulty, marking is carried out by using the marking key provided. The child reads the passages silently and then writes in the missing word. The subject is not penalised for incorrect spelling. One point is awarded for each correct response. The total test score is then converted into a reading age. The two forms B and R are parallel tests which augment rather than duplicate each other.

GAPADOL *Reading Comprehension Test* by J. McLeod and J. Anderson (1987) is the equivalent of the above for adolescents.

London Reading Test (1978)

Age range
Children from 10;7 to 12;4 years. It may also be suitable for adults who are experiencing difficulties with reading

[Developed by a group of teachers and researchers working in inner London.]

Aims/Purpose
This test was designed specifically for use in ethnically diverse areas and may be used as a survey/screening test when children are preparing to transfer from primary to secondary education.

Materials
There is a small manual, practice sheets A and B, and record forms A and B.

Time taken
It is not a timed test, but could take up to an hour

Publisher/Distributor
NFER-Nelson

Administration
The forms contain three passages at a level of difficulty similar to that of text books commonly used in the first year of secondary education. The first two passages require that the subject fills in the correct word. The third passage has a series of questions about its content. The passages have been specifically written to reduce bias against children from multicultural backgrounds. It may be administered in a group. It is possible to use the third passage with adults. The tests provide detailed information about the child's level of reading attainment and pattern of abilities. Results indicate whether the subject can cope with material without the aid of a teacher and highlight if remedial help may be needed in the secondary school.

Macmillan Individual Reading Analysis (MIRA) (1990)

Authors
D. Vincent and
M. de la Mare

Consultant:
H. Arnold

Age range
Children from 5 to 10 years

Time taken
It is not a timed test

Publisher/Distributor
Macmillan Education

Aims/Purpose
MIRA assesses the standards and progress of children who are having difficulties in learning to read.

Materials
There is an administration manual, three parallel series of reading booklets and corresponding record sheets. A book *Teacher's Guide to Individual Reading Analysis* is also available.

Administration
This test complements the *New Macmillan Reading Analysis* (see page 70) at the lower end of the scale as it is particularly sensitive to the early stages of reading. It is individually administered. There are three parallel series of reading booklets: X, Y and Z, each containing five graded reading passages. Results yield a specific reading age, and offer a diagnostic analysis of reading strategies, including miscue analysis. The test provides scores for both accuracy and comprehension for children from approximately 5;7 to 10;6 years of age. It has been standardised in the UK. Further diagnostic details, and analysis and details regarding the development of the test, are described in the book.

National Adult Reading Test (NART) (1982)

Author
H.E. Nelson

Age range
Adults from 20 to 70 years

Time taken
It is not a timed test

Publisher/Distributor
NFER-Nelson

Aims/Purpose
This test was designed to provide a means of estimating the pre-morbid intelligence levels of adult clients suspected of suffering from intellectual deterioration. It may be useful in measuring the effect of drugs, alcohol, illness and psychiatric problems on the client's level of intellectual function.

Materials
The kit consists of a soft-backed manual, word cards and score sheets.

Administration
The test comprises a list of 50 words printed in order of increasing difficulty. The words are relatively short to avoid the possible adverse effects of stimulus complexity on the reading of clients who are suffering from dementia. The words are all irregular with respect to pronunciation to minimise the possibility of reading by phonemic decoding rather than word recognition. WAIS, verbal performance and full scale IQs may be predicted from the score obtained. The test was standardised on 120 patients with extracerebral disorders, mainly spinal cord disorders and peripheral neuropathies. A detailed validation is given.

Neale Analysis of Reading Ability – Revised British edition (1989)

Author
M.D. Neale

British adaptation
U. Christophers and C. Whetton

Age range
Children from 5 to 13 years

[This replaces the *Neale Analysis of Reading Ability* by N.B. Neale (1981).]

Aims/Purpose
The aims of this test are to measure the accuracy, rate and comprehension level of children's reading, in order to enable teachers to plan appropriate teaching programmes for individual children.

Materials
A plastic wallet contains the manual, reader, demonstration audio cassette, record forms one and two, and diagnostic tutor record forms. A tape-recorder will be required.

Time taken
It is not a timed test but takes about 20 minutes

Publisher/Distributor
NFER-Nelson

Administration
The test should be administered individually. It is in three forms. Forms 1 and 2 are standardised and each contains six passages. The Diagnostic Tutor Form contains ten graded passages and an extension passage for more advanced readers. It also includes additional passages at the upper and lower ability levels which help to identify children with special needs. The Diagnostic Tutor Form may be used as the basis for miscue analysis as well as criterion-referenced and diagnostic assessment. The test passage is presented in an illustrated colour-coded reader. The correspondingly colour-coded record forms enable the assessor to record: an analysis of errors as each passage is read, the time taken, and the answers to the comprehension sections. This new British edition has been revised and re-standardised.

New Macmillan Reading Analysis (1986)

Authors
D. Vincent and
M. de la Mare

Consultant
H. Arnold

Age range
Children from 7 to 11+ years. It may also be suitable for adults who are experiencing difficulties reading

Time taken
It is not a timed test

Publisher/Distributor
Macmillan Education

Aims/Purpose
The test assesses the reading standards and progress of older children. It is an oral test which may be used for long-term monitoring.

Materials
There is a manual, three parallel series of reading booklets and corresponding record forms.

Administration
This is an oral test which is administered individually. A child reads aloud up to six graded passages, and then orally answers questions on each passage. There are three parallel sets of passages: A, B and C, which allows for re-testing and monitoring of progress. The material has been carefully selected to be appropriate for older children and adults. The graded passages allow clinical and diagnostic analysis of reading strategies, including miscue analysis, and types of errors may be classified on the record sheets. There are standardised norms provided for accuracy and comprehension for children from 7 to 12 years.

Assessing Reading Difficulties – second edition (1984) A Diagnostic and Remedial Approach

Author
L. Bradley

Age range
Children from 5 to 12 years who need remedial help. Because of its auditory nature, it may also be used with younger children

Time taken
It is not timed, but is 'short'

Publisher/Distributor
Macmillan Education

Aims/Purpose
The test aims to assess a child's rhyming abilities and to offer remedial help based on the findings. It is for use by teachers and therapists as a diagnostic schedule, for children who are making little progress learning to read.

Materials
A paperback manual and test sheets.

Administration
This test is simple to administer. It is an auditory test, requiring the child to identify rhyming words from four words read aloud by the assessor. The author's research has shown that training in rhyming may lead to improvement in reading, and suggestions for remediation are included in the book.

Diagnostic Spelling Test (1982)

Authors
D. Vincent and J. Claydon

Age range
Mostly children from 7;8 to 11;8 years, although it may be used with older children who are known to have spelling difficulties

Time taken
It is untimed. It is suitable for group administration and time may be allowed for less able spellers to attempt all items

Publisher/Distributor
NFER-Nelson

Aims/Purpose
It is designed to identify reliably and diagnose spelling difficulties among groups of children or individual children. It appraises the severity of the difficulties and indicates directions which practical remediation work may take.

Materials
The test consists of a teacher's manual and pupil's booklet and record form.

Administration
There are seven subtests which may be completed directly on the form:
(1) homophones
(2) common words
(3) proofreading letter strings
(4) nonsense words
(5) dictionary use
(6) self-concept
(7) dictation is also part of the test and this may be given separately.

Two sets of forms, A and B, are available so that subjects

may be re-tested to mark progress on similar but not identical items. The material on both forms has been standardised and tables are provided in the manual for conversion of raw scores to a standardised score scale. The test is particularly discriminating among below-average spellers.

SEVERE LEARNING DIFFICULTIES

Affective Communication Assessment (ACA) (1985)

Authors
J. Coupe, L. Barton, M. Barber, L. Collins, D. Levy and D. Murphy

Age range
Children with severe learning difficulties who are at an early stage of sensorimotor development

Time taken
It is not a timed assessment, it may be administered over an extended period of time

Publisher/Distributor
Special Education Resource Centre

Aims/Purpose
The ACA was developed by teachers as an assessment tool for teachers, speech and language therapists and other professionals working with developmentally delayed or handicapped children. It is an observation schedule, focusing on pre-intentional communication skills and communicative behaviours. These behaviours are observed and interpreted so that predictions may be made regarding the child's repertoire of affective communication. Based on the information gathered, appropriate intervention may then be planned, which will reinforce and strengthen potentially communicative signals.

Materials
ACA is a slim soft-backed book containing recording sheets for the three component areas of the assessment as well as details regarding administration and scoring.

Administration
There are three component areas of the assessment:
1. *Observation:* beginning with familiar situations, the teacher observes and records the child's positive and negative responses to a wide range of stimuli. These may be auditory, visual, olfactory, tactile, taste or environmental. The meaning of these responses is interpreted, e.g. likes/does not like.
2. *Identification:* the pattern of frequency and consistency of these responses is recorded.
3. *Intervention:* from the information accumulated on the recording sheets, intervention may be planned, to encourage and increase communicative and potentially communicative behaviours.

Is This Autism? (1987)

Authors
M. Aarons and
T. Gittens

Age range
Children, mostly
from 2 to 8 years

Time taken
It is not a timed
assessment

Publisher/Distributor
NFER-Nelson

Aims/Purpose
This checklist is for use by speech and language therapists or any professionals working with children who present autistic features. It aims to help the assessor gather information which will identify the child's developmental level, and help to define appropriate and realistic intervention. This is achieved by placing a child on a continuum of social/educational language deficit, rather than providing a diagnostic label.

Materials
There is a soft-backed handbook and checklist.

Administration
The section headings in the handbook and checklist are cross-referred. The handbook includes general information regarding autism as well as exploring the details of the checklist. The checklist is divided into eight sections:
(1) general observation (including appearance, movement, behaviour, sociability and management)
(2) attention control (six stages)
(3) sensory function
(4) non-verbal symbolic function
(5) concept formation
(6) sequencing and rhythmic abilities
(7) speech and language
(8) educational attainment and intelligence.
Information from these sections may be collated to provide a profile of the child's strengths and weaknesses which should help to identify the child's developmental level and provide a working basis for treatment planning. Appropriate age levels for many of the behaviours are indicated.

Behaviour Assessment Battery (1982)

Authors
C. Kiernan and
M. Jones

Aims/Purpose
It may be used for assessment, detailed goal planning and evaluation. It aims to help the care worker find teaching targets for profoundly handicapped people, in a variety of areas. Some sections are suitable for use with blind, deaf and physically handicapped people.

Age range
For use with people with severe learning difficulties, particularly useful with children

Time taken
It is not a timed assessment and may be used over an extended period

Publisher/Distributor
NFER-Nelson

Materials
All the information is provided in a paperbacked book. However, the assessment makes use of a large amount of material which is not provided and must be assembled by the assessor.

Administration
Each area covered has its own score sheet (lattice) with subgroups arranged developmentally from left to right, whereas the items within the subgroups are arranged in order of difficulty from top to bottom. Boxes are ticked as steps are achieved, showing a visual profile of progress. The areas covered are: reinforcement and experience; inspection; tracking; visuomotor; auditory; postural control; exploratory play; constructive play; search strategies; perceptual problem solving; social; communication, including sign language; self-help skills. A summary of each item is written in a box on the score sheet.

The Communication Assessment Profile for Adults with a Mental Handicap (CASP) (1988)

Author
A. van der Gaag

Age range
Adults with severe-to-mild learning difficulties

Time taken
Carer's assessment takes 15 minutes. Therapist's/joint assessment takes 30–45 minutes (this may be ongoing over several sessions)

Publisher
Speech Profiles

Distributors
Speech Profiles
Winslow Press

Aims/Purpose
CASP examines the communicative abilities of adults with learning difficulties in everyday situations and within their own communication environments. Administered jointly by care staff and speech and language therapists, it aims to give a descriptive screening assessment of the client's communication skills, understanding and expression of speech and language.

Materials/Administration
CASP consists of three assessments.
1. *Carer's assessment:* this comprises a questionnaire. Section 1 presents 33 questions relating to the client's communicative abilities. Four further questions in Section 2 are related to the client's specific home environment.
2. *Therapist's assessment:* the eight sections of subtests include: event knowledge; hearing and auditory skills; vocabulary; comprehension (objects, sentences); communicative functions; and expressive skills. Four additional appendices cover: concepts; articulation; imitation of gesture, and oromuscular skills.
3. *Joint assessment:* this summary of assessment includes the client's own views, client's strengths, profile sum-

mary, a communication environment rating scale, and priorities for change.

CASP is primarily a descriptive assessment and percentile rankings of the raw scores achieved on the subtests may be plotted to give a profile of the client's communicative abilities. These rankings are based on a sample of mentally handicapped adults. Priorities for change are discussed based on a 'strengths and weaknesses' model.

The Communication Schedule (1975)

Author
K. Mogford

Age range
Young children with learning difficulties; pre-verbal children with profound learning disabilities

Time taken
It is not timed

Publisher/Distributor
Child Development Research Unit, University of Nottingham

Aims/Purpose
It is intended that the schedule be used with parents of young children with learning difficulties, as a guide for probing and questioning. Responses may help therapists in planning their counselling approach.

Materials
The schedule consists of typewritten sheets of questions.

Administration
Originally designed for a professionally run toy library, the data gleaned from such probing are designed to give a profile of the child's functional communication skills. Initial questions relate mainly to information for research purposes, whilst the remainder are intended to assess pre-verbal levels of the child's natural communication for parent/professional remediative partnerships, and to open up areas for discussion regarding management of the child. There are no normative data. It has been recommended by Mark Masidlover for children below the level addressed by the Derbyshire Language Scheme (see below).

The Derbyshire Language Scheme – Revised edition (DLS) (1982)

Authors
W. Knowles and M. Masidlover

Aims/Purpose
The scheme aims to assess the level of language functioning, in terms of both comprehension and expression, and to make recommendations about approaches to language teaching based on the assessment. The scheme may be used by professionals working with children across all levels of learning difficulties, as well as with language-delayed and pre-school children. A screening test is available for use with adults with severe learning difficulties.

Age range
Specifically it is for children and adults with learning difficulties, although it may be used with children with speech and language difficulties

Time taken
The tests are untimed and may be recorded over several sessions

Publisher/Distributor
Mark Masidlover, Derbyshire Education Authority

Materials
The scheme consists of four large ringbinders: user's manual, picture test manual, and two teaching manuals. There are specific forms for recording assessment results and progress: Rapid Screening Test; Detailed Test of Comprehension; Progress Record Form, Assessment Summary.

Administration
The Rapid Screening Test establishes the level at which more detailed assessment of comprehension should proceed. Assessment of comprehension begins at the one-word level and progresses in logical sequence to include negatives, questions, verbs, pronouns, articles, prepositions and conjunctions. The assessment of comprehension is based on the number of information-carrying words (ICW). The test makes use of both toys and pictures for assessment purposes. Expressive language is assessed in as natural a setting as possible and is elicited during the assessment of comprehension. The toys are not included in the kit as it is intended that age-appropriate and person-appropriate materials should be used for assessment. The assessment is not standardised and there are no age equivalents.

(A training course must be completed prior to purchasing the materials.)

ENABLE – Encouraging a Natural and Better Life Experience (1990)

Authors
L.H. Brown and A. Keens

Age range
Adults with learning difficulties

Time taken
It is not timed

Publisher/Distributor
Forum Consultancy

Aims/Purpose
ENABLE is a systematic approach to the facilitation of the functional communication skills of adults with learning difficulties. It is an intervention approach, incorporating an assessment schedule, a programme planner and a resource section.

Materials
A binder contains all the relevant material.

Administration
ENABLE is divided into four sections:
1. *Training schedule* for use with carers who are to be involved in implementing the ENABLE approach.
2. *Profile section* which provides a summary of the formal and informal assessments made by the speech and language therapists and the carers. This is not an assessment in itself, but provides a structured way of summarising information on the clients and their com-

munication environment.
3. *Programme section* which provides the details of intervention for each client on three levels: individual, group, and environment. Specific targets for intervention are worked out by the speech and language therapist and carer, using a goal plan approach.
4. *Resource section* which consists of step-by-step guidelines on how communication skills can be taught on an individual, group and environment level.
General and specific intervention techniques are described in detail in this section.

INTECOM (1990)

Author
S. Jones

Age range
Adults with learning difficulties

Time taken
This is not specified

Publisher/Distributor
NFER-Nelson

Aims/Purpose
INTECOM is a package designed to INTEgrate carers into the assessment and development of COMmunication skills in people with learning difficulties. Its primary focus is on changing the individual's communication environment – specifically the nature and scope of relationships, and the opportunities which the individual has for communicating on a day-to-day basis.

Materials
A ringbinder contains all the necessary materials and forms.

Administration
INTECOM consists of three sections. The first is a *training package* for use with carers. This pack contains guidelines and materials for running five workshops on communication. They are designed to allow carers to explore their own perceptions of communication, and to look at how these influence the way they communicate with their clients. The second is *opportunity planning*. In this section, carers are asked to identify those aspects of the environment which are preventing clients from using their communication skills to the fullest extent. Having identified these, strategies for overcoming environmental constraints are developed. The third section is a *communication checklist* which allows the carer to record how the client is communicating. It summarises various aspects of communication, such as motivation, level of expressive language, intelligibility and clarity. It also provides a summary of the carer's perception of how the client is using his or her communication on a day-to-day basis.

The Interaction Checklist for Augmentative Communication (INCH) (1984)

Authors
S.O. Bolton and
S.E. Dashiell

Age range
Unspecified

Distributors
IMAGINART
Communication
Products, USA
Winslow Press

Aims/Purpose
INCH is an observational checklist which may be used in the evaluation and remediation of the interactive skills of non-speaking clients. It aims to describe the critical features of interactions between augmentative system users and their interlocutors, and to facilitate the formulation of goals and objectives for clinical intervention.

Materials
INCH comprises a slim ring-bound manual and separate checklist sheets.

Administration
The observed behaviours are recorded on individual sheets. This information includes: the client's ability to initiate, facilitate, regulate and terminate communicative interactions, using an augmentative system. The client is considered both as a sender and as a receiver of messages. The recorded data may be used as an initial measure of communicative effectiveness with an electronic device or manual system and progress may be followed up and recorded on the summary charts. Suggestions for teaching strategies are included in the manual.

Personal Communication Plan (PCP) (1991)

Authors
A. Hitchings and
R. Spence

Age range
From 14 years to adult

Time taken
This may vary as it is a long-term assessment and programme plan

Publisher/Distributor
NFER-Nelson

Aims/Purpose
The PCP is designed to assess the functional communication skills and environmental opportunities of people with mild-to-severe learning disabilities. It aims to involve as many people as possible who are relevant to the client's everyday environment.

Materials
A plastic folder contains the manual and checklist booklets.

Administration
The PCP has been 'structured within the framework of the five accomplishments of normalisation'. It is divided into five sections:

(1) background information
(2) speech and language skills
(3) social communication skills
(4) environment
(5) shared action planning.

The first four sections comprise the assessment of the client's expressed communication, as well as considering the communicative environment which may be affecting the client's motivation and effectiveness in communicating. The section on shared action planning then allows for goals to be set which aim to improve the client's abilities and opportunities for communication within his or her environment.

Pre-feeding Skills (1987)

Authors
S. Evans Morris and
M. Dunn Klein

Age range
Very young children, or older children with profound feeding difficulties

Time taken
This is intended to be used for on-going assessment

Publisher
Therapy Skill Builders

Distributor
Winslow Press

Aims/Purpose
The aim of this book is to provide a comprehensive resource for feeding development. It aims to encourage clinicians to examine different ways of thinking and learning about the assessment and treatment of young children with feeding difficulties.

Materials
A thick spirally bound volume with soft covers.

Administration
There are 20 chapters which are subdivided and cover: anatomy and physiology of the oral–pharyngeal structure; assessment; approaches to treatment; the environment (in relation to feeding); nutrition; speech and communication (in relation to feeding); pre-feeding issues specific to different groups of children (e.g. blind, cleft palate); materials; individual planning. The sections are illustrated by cartoon drawings and are clearly laid out in subsections. Several options are offered for solving some of the problems raised. Each chapter includes: probes; self-regulating questions; participation experiences to encourage the clinician actively to test potential solutions; resource lists; and reproducible assessment charts and checklists.

Pre-symbol Assessment (1979)

Authors
Blissymbolics Communications Resource Centre

Age range
Not specified; may be used with anyone with difficulties in expressive communication

Time taken
It is not a timed assessment

Distributors
Blissymbolics Communications (UK) Resource Centre
Winslow Press

Aims/Purpose
The assessment aims to provide guidelines regarding the appropriateness of introducing a symbols system to a non-verbal client (with specific reference to Blissymbols).

Materials
It is a small spirally bound book.

Administration
The book contains symbol drawings and instructions for administration and some score forms. It is not a standardised test, but may be used as a screening device. It takes a visual–perceptual approach in trying to determine whether a child or adult can relate to, and ultimately recognise, symbols. It is based on six developmental stages in relation to visual materials. The manual is divided into six sections so that the developmental level of the potential user may be determined.

Pre-verbal Communication Schedule (PVCS) (1987)

Authors
C. Kiernan and B. Reid

Age range
Children or adults with severe learning difficulties. It may also be used with normally developing infants, non-speaking deaf children and people with severe physical handicaps

Aims/Purpose
This checklist is designed to assess the communication skills of people who do not speak or who have little expressive language: words, signs or symbols. It provides a detailed profile of their pre-communicative, communicative and receptive skills, and provides data to help staff develop individual communication programmes.

Materials
The Schedule comprises a manual, checklist and scoring sheets in a plastic folder. There is a photocopy master of a programme planning sheet which may be used to record the progress of individual clients.

Administration
The 195 items on the checklist are divided into four main sections:

Time taken
The full schedule may take an hour to complete. The shortened version takes approximately 35 minutes

Publisher/Distributor
NFER-Nelson

(1) pre-communicative
(2) informal communication skills
(3) formal communication skills
(4) receptive skills.

These are further divided into subsections. A summary score sheet enables areas of strengths and weaknesses to be identified. The manual provides detailed instructions and suggests how the interpretation of the scores may lead to appropriate intervention. A shortened form of the Schedule provides data to aid functional communication programme planning. The full version includes additional details regarding pre-communicative behaviour.

A Clinical and Educational Manual for Use with the *Uzgiris and Hunt Scales of Infant Psychological Development* (1980)

Author
C.J. Dunst

Age range
Infants or young children with delayed development

Time taken
This is not a timed procedure

Publisher/Distributor
PRO-ED, USA

Aims/Purpose
This manual is based on *Assessment in Infancy: Ordinal Scales of Psychological Development* (1975) by I.C. Uzgiris and J.McV. Hunt, published by University of Illinois Press. It aims to translate these scales into procedural guidelines which may be used to determine an individual's overall pattern of sensorimotor development.

Materials
There is a large format illustrated paperback book, and scoring forms. These include: summary record forms; profile of abilities forms; and individual scale record forms.

Administration
There are four sections in the manual: introduction; general description of the record forms; directions for administering and scoring; recording, profiling and interpreting the results. The procedures are designed to give insight into the child's sensorimotor abilities, and thus to facilitate the design of activities for appropriate intervention.

VISION

Developmental Test of Visual Perception – Revised edition (1964)

Author
M. Frostig

Age range
Children from 3 to 8 years, although it may be used with older children with learning difficulties, and may also be useful with adults with aphasia

Time taken
It is untimed, although it takes approximately 30–40 minutes

Publisher
Consulting Psychologists Press Inc., USA

Distributor
Oxford Psychologists Press

Aims/Purpose
The test can be used as a screening device for young children and as a clinical evaluative instrument for older children with learning difficulties.

Materials
There is a manual, monograph, test booklets, demonstration cards and scoring keys. Coloured pencils are also required but are not provided.

Administration
Subtests, each containing several items measure five areas of perceptual skills:
(1) eye–motor coordination
(2) figure–ground
(3) constancy of shape
(4) position in space
(5) spatial relationships
so that a child's visual–perceptual disabilities may be discovered as early as possible.

It may be administered to an individual or to a group. Raw scores can be translated into perceptual age equivalents and scaled scores for each subtest. A perceptual quotient can be computed. The manual and monograph include information regarding reliability and validity studies.

Stycar Vision Tests (1976)

Author
M. Sheridan

Age range
Children from 6 months to 7 years

Time taken
It is not a timed test

Publisher/Distributor
NFER-Nelson

Aims/Purpose
The aim is to test and record a child's overall visual competence. The tests are divided into three different age groups: infants, pre-school and school entrants. It may also be used with children with severe learning difficulties with a corresponding mental age. A fourth test may be used for older children with more severe visual or multiple handicaps.

Materials
A box contains toys, charts, test aids and record forms for all four tests, as well as the revised manual.

Administration
Infants from 6 months to 2;6 years are tested on their ability to follow moving objects, fix on a static object, perceive movement in the peripheral fields, and voluntarily attend to a visual stimulus. This test may also be used with children who have motor difficulties, learning difficulties and expressive language problems. *Pre-school children* are required to match key letters on cards with a chart, and name some miniature toys. For *school-aged children* from 5 to 7 years, their vision is assessed in each eye as they draw letters. *The Panda Test* is a matching test for children from 5 to 15 months with acute visual and/or multiple handicaps. The results offer a comprehensive assessment of a child's visual competence.

Part IV

Tests associated with acquired disorders

Aphasia

An Aphasia Screening Test 88
R. Whurr

The Assessment of Aphasia and Related Disorders – second edition
Incorporating: The Boston Diagnostic Aphasia Examination –
Revised; and The Boston Naming Test 89
H. Goodglass, E. Kaplan and S. Weintraub

The Children's Aphasia Screening Test 90
R. Whurr and S. Evans

Examining for Aphasia – Revised edition 91
J. Eisenson

Communicative Abilities in Daily Living (CADL) 91
A.L. Holland

Revised Edinburgh Functional Communication Profile (EFCP) 92
S:L. Wirz, C. Skinner and E. Dean

Frenchay Aphasia Screening Test (FAST) 93
P. Enderby, V. Wood and D. Wade

The Functional Communication Profile 94
M.T. Sarno

Graded Naming Test 95
P. McKenna and E. Warrington

Minnesota Test for Differential Diagnosis of Aphasia – Revised edition 95
H. Schuell

Shortened Form of the Minnesota Test for Differential
Diagnosis of Aphasia 96
J. Thompson and P. Enderby

Contributions to Neuropsychological Assessment 97
A.L. Benton, K. Hamsher, N. Varney and O. Spreen

The Neurosensory Centre Comprehensive Examination for Aphasia 98
O. Spreen and A.L. Benton

Porch Index of Communicative Ability (PICA) 99
B.E. Porch

Psycholinguistic Assessments of Language Processing
in Aphasia (PALPA) 99
J. Kay, R. Lesser and M. Coltheart

The Right Hemisphere Language Battery 100
K.L. Bryan

The Token Test 101
E. de Renzi and L.A. Vignolo

Revised Token Test 102
M.M. McNeil and T.E. Prescott

The Western Aphasia Battery (WAB) 102
A. Kertesz

Apraxia

Apraxia Battery for Adults (ABA) 103
B.L. Dabul

Degenerative disorder

Anomalous Sentences Repetition Test 104
D. Weeks

Dysphasia/Dementia Screening Test 104
A.M. Phillips

The Kendrick Cognitive Tests for the Elderly 105
D. Kendrick

Dysarthria

Frenchay Dysarthria Assessment and Computer Differential Analysis –
second edition 106
P. Enderby

Robertson Dysarthria Profile 107
S.J. Robertson

Dysphagia

Dysphagia Care with Acute and Long-term Patients 107
N. O'Sullivan

APHASIA

An Aphasia Screening Test (1974)

Author
R. Whurr

Age range
Adults who have suffered brain damage

Time taken
It is not a timed test

Publisher/Distributor
Whurr Publishers

Aims/Purpose
This is a short, simple but sensitive screening tool which aims to identify language disturbances (listening, speaking, reading and writing) in brain-damaged adults who demonstrate a moderate-to-severe impairment of communication skills. It is not suitable for minimally impaired aphasic people.

Materials
A manual, display books, test cards, test objects, record forms, transcription forms and writing booklets are provided in a lightweight plastic folder.

Administration
There are 50 short subtests each consisting of five items: 20 for receptive function; 28 for expressive function; and 2 for calculation. Within the receptive category there are four 'pre-assessment' tests to screen for severe visual perceptual disorders; eight reading tests, both visual matching and comprehension; and eight auditory language tests, selecting on command: pictures, colours, numbers, letters, words and sentences, and carrying out simple and complex oral commands. Within the expressive category are speech (articulation) tests, naming tests, tests of descriptive ability and writing tests. A profile of the subject's performance can be plotted, thus showing clearly their successes and failures. Raw scores may be objectively categorised into one of six groups, ranging from 'no defects' to 'very severe defects'. The manual also contains 14 case histories illustrating use of the test.

The Assessment of Aphasia and Related Disorders – second edition (1983)

This complete package comprises *The Boston Diagnostic Aphasia Examination* and *The Boston Naming Test*.

The Boston Diagnostic Aphasia Examination – Revised edition (1983)

Authors
H. Goodglass and
E. Kaplan

Age range
Adult aphasic patients

Time taken
It is not a timed test

Aims/Purpose
This test aims to diagnose the type of aphasic syndrome present and to measure the level of performance over a wide range of abilities. It provides a comprehensive assessment of the assets and liabilities of the patient in all language areas so that appropriate therapy may be applied.

Materials
A test manual, test booklets, including appropriate text and test cards showing stimulus material are available. (This is part of a complete package – see above.)

Administration
The tests were devised in order to elicit quantitative evidence of the area of deficit. Where objective quantification is not possible, rating scales are provided. The language tests include detailed assessment of: conversational and expository speech; auditory comprehension; oral expression, understanding of written language; and writing. Scores can be used to plot profiles. The detailed text includes chapters on the nature of aphasic disorders, details of the test procedures to supplement the test manual, and descriptions of the major aphasic syndromes and their expected test profiles/patterns. There are supplementary language tests which include the exploration of psycholinguistic factors in auditory comprehension and expression, and the screening for hemispheric disconnection symptoms. Supplementary non-language tests include tests for constructional apraxia, finger agnosia, acalculia and right/left confusion. The scores are given as a percentile ranking.

The Boston Naming Test (1983)

Authors
H. Goodglass,
E. Kaplan and
S. Weintraub

Age range
Children and adults

Publisher
Lea and Febiger,
Philadelphia, USA

Distributor
Williams & Wilkins

Aims/Purpose
This is a wide range naming vocabulary test. It may be used in the assessment of children with learning difficulties in addition to being a supplement to the Boston Diagnostic Aphasia Examination for aphasic adults.

Materials
The test comprises a book of stimulus material (60 pictures) and a test booklet. (Available as part of the complete package – see above.)

Administration
Latency is measured and the patient's response is recorded verbatim. Stimulus cues and/or phonemic cues are given in the event of a failed response. Approximate norms are available for children, aged 5;6 to 10;6 years, normal adults and adults with aphasia.

The Children's Aphasia Screening Test (1986)

Authors
R. Whurr and
S. Evans

Age range
Children, no age specified

Time taken
Untimed, but 'short'

Publisher/Distributor
Whurr Publishers

Aims/Purpose
This is a short screening test which aims to provide a profile of the communication processes: listening; comprehension; speech; pre-reading; writing; and gesture. This may be used to identify language disturbance in the brain-damaged child who has an acquired moderate-to-severe impairment of language function. The profile may also prove helpful in planning treatment.

Materials
A ringbinder contains a display book and manual, test objects and cards. Record forms, transcription forms and drawing forms are also included.

Administration
There are 25 subtests, 12 of receptive and 13 of expressive function. Receptive subtests include: tests of visual perception; a pre-reading test; and auditory language tests. The expressive category includes four pre-speech tests, and six expressive language tests including: naming, sentence formulation, picture description, and conversational responses. Two drawing tests and a gestural test are also included. A profile of performance may be plotted on the

summary record form. The manual contains the results of the normative data collated from a sample of pre-school and school-age children from 3 to 7 years. The results yielded are quantitative as well as qualitative and are easy to interpret.

Examining for Aphasia – Revised edition (1954)

Author
J. Eisenson

Age range
Primarily for use with adolescents and adults with acquired aphasia, but it can be used with 'congenital aphasics'

Time taken
It is an untimed assessment, dependent on the patient

Publisher
Harcourt Brace Jovanovich

Distributor
The Psychological Corporation

Aims/Purpose
The aims are to provide a guided approach for evaluating aphasic language disturbances and other disturbances closely related to language function, such as agnosias and apraxias: to reveal both the assets and the deficits of the patient and the degree, as well as the areas, of dysfunction. The test can be used for screening purposes by reducing the number of items used.

Materials
A manual containing stimulus pictures and words, and 12-page record forms are provided. Some common objects are also needed.

Administration
The assessment is divided into two main areas: receptive and expressive. Items include: visual and/or tactile and/or oral recognition of objects; pictures; colours; numbers; letters; words; comprehension of sentences; reading comprehension; imitation of actions; use of gesture; repetition of numbers; words and sentences; naming; spelling and simple arithmetic. Results are analysed qualitatively. The manual contains several chapters on aphasia and related problems as well as details of the administration of the test and interpretation of the results. This is a standardised procedure (USA).

Communicative Abilities in Daily Living (CADL) (1980) A test of functional communication for aphasic adults

Author
A.L. Holland

Age range
Adults with aphasia

Aims/Purpose
The CADL was designed as a supplementary tool to enable professionals working with aphasic adults to assess the functional communication skills of their patients.

Time taken
This is not a timed assessment

Publisher
PRO-ED, USA

Distributor
Taskmaster Ltd

Materials
The kit is contained in a sturdy box and includes: an administration manual, including detailed instructions; a scoring kit of scoring booklets with a prescription envelope, pad of appointment cards and pad of patient forms; a spiral-bound colour picture book; and a 30-minute training audio-cassette tape, with the four auditory stimuli necessary for testing. A tape-recorder will be required.

Administration
The test covers 10 categories:
(1) reading/writing/calculating
(2) speech acts
(3) content utilisation
(4) role playing
(5) sequential relationships
(6) social conventions
(7) divergences
(8) non-verbal symbols
(9) deixis (movement-related communicative behaviour)
(10) humour, metaphor and absurdity.

The administration of the test is a combination of orthodox testing and role-playing. Descriptive data are gathered in each of the categories so that a profile of the patient's strengths and weaknesses is compiled. This may then be used to help plan a treatment and management programme. The test provides cut-off scores for determining functional communication disorders. Normative data have been collated in the USA using normal and aphasic adults.

Revised Edinburgh Functional Communication Profile (EFCP) (1990)

Authors
S.L. Wirz,
C. Skinner and
E. Dean

Age range
Adults with aphasia, traumatic head injury, physical handicaps and developmental delays, and children with developmental language disorders

[This replaces the *Edinburgh Functional Communication Profile* (1984) by C. Skinner, S. Wirz, I. Thompson and J. Davidson distributed by Winslow Press.]

Aims/Purpose
The profile was designed to structure the observation and analysis of an individual's communicative functioning. It was designed to supplement traditional assessments by providing important information about an individual's ability to use linguistic skills in particular contexts. It gives pragmatic information essential to the development of effective management and intervention programmes.

Time taken
The assessment is untimed

Publisher/Distributor
Communication Skill Builders, USA

Materials
The profile consists of a manual and assessment forms, enclosed in a plastic wallet.

Administration
The EFCP provides two profiles of the client's ability to interact: the Interaction Analysis and the Communicative Performance Analysis. The profile assesses two parameters: the ability to engage in and sustain interaction; and the verbal and non-verbal modalities used to achieve communication. Efficacy rating of the *Interaction Analysis* is based on 10 conversational exchanges. The communicative functions included in the *Communicative Performance Analysis* are: greeting; acknowledging; responding; requesting; and initiating. The modalities for communication include: speech, gesture, writing, facial expression and vocalisation. Efficacy in these functions is recorded on the assessment forms. A supplementary interview provides suggested protocols for eliciting communicative intent that are not observed in spontaneous conversation.

Frenchay Aphasia Screening Test (FAST) (1987)

Authors
P. Enderby, V. Wood and D. Wade

Age range
Adults

Time taken
Three to 10 minutes

Publisher/Distributor
NFER-Nelson

Aims/Purpose
FAST is meant to be used as a quick standardised screening device by any professional concerned with adult aphasia and left hemisphere brain damage. The test assesses comprehension and expression of language, reading and writing, and may be used to aid diagnosis in initial assessment.

Materials
The pack consists of a manual, a picture card and record forms.

Administration
The client is asked to identify some illustrated shapes and to answer questions about the composite picture which is presented. Five graded written sentences are used as further stimulus items. Peel-off record forms are used for scoring. The test has been standardised in the UK and cut-off scores for the client's age level, based on studies of over 120 normal adults, are given.

The Functional Communication Profile (1969)

Author
M.T. Sarno

Age range
Primarily for use with adults with aphasia, but can be used with children

Time taken
It is not a timed test

Publisher
New York University Medical Center, USA

Distributor
Educational Center, New York University Medical Center, USA

Aims/Purpose
The profile is a standardised rating scale which aims to quantify the communication behaviours the patient uses when interacting with others. It aims to assess the use the patient/client makes of residual communication skills which may or may not be apparent on clinical testing of the language impairment. The profile should be used in conjunction with tests assessing clinical performance.

Materials
Manual and test forms are provided.

Administration
The test form details 45 communication behaviours in everyday life; each behaviour is rated on a 9-point scale on the basis of non-structured conversation with the patient and observation, for example, of reading. The scale ranges from 'normal ability' (100%) to 'absent ability' (0%) and the functional abilities measured include: indicating yes/no; reading newspaper headlines; making change. All degrees of severity can be measured, including the performance of the non-speaking patient who uses gesture. The items are grouped under five headings:
(1) movement
(2) speaking
(3) understanding
(4) reading
(5) miscellaneous, which includes calculation and writing.

The manual contains details of the expected response, suggestions for conversation, details of rating and scoring and guidelines on interpretation. Performance is indexed relative to the patient's estimated pre-morbid level of communicative ability. 'Normal' is defined by the clinician's skilled estimation so that the profile is designed for use only by those experienced clinicians who have experience with many aphasic patients. Use by an inexperienced clinician may invalidate the result.

Graded Naming Test (1983)

Authors
P. McKenna and
E. Warrington

Age range
Adults

Time taken
It is an untimed test

Publisher/Distributor
NFER-Nelson

Aims/Purpose
This test may be used with any adult. It aims to test the subject's naming ability and to detect a mild impairment of language function.

Materials
The test materials consist of a manual, an object picture booklet and record sheets.

Administration
The test comprises 30 black-and-white line drawings which the subject is asked to name. The vocabulary is carefully graded in order of difficulty and ranges from words such as 'kangaroo' and 'buoy' to words such as 'cowl' and 'retort'. Equivalent scores on *WAIS Vocabulary*, *National Adult Reading Test* and *Schonell Graded Word Reading Test* can be devised from a conversion table. The test was standardised in the UK on normal volunteers and extracerebrally disordered adults between 20 and 76 years of age. Raw scores are calculated and these may be interpreted by drawing comparisons with the subjects' estimated pre-morbid vocabulary.

Minnesota Test for Differential Diagnosis of Aphasia – Revised edition (1973)

Author
H. Schuell

Age range
Adults with aphasia

Time taken
This is not a timed test

Publisher/Distributor
NFER-Nelson

Aims/Purpose
Through this test the therapist may observe the level at which language performance breaks down in each of the principal language modalities. It aims to pinpoint the processes which underlie this breakdown, thus enabling differential diagnosis into one of the five major or two minor categories identified by the test.

Materials
The test comprises stimulus cards, the administrative manual, and the Monograph: *Different Diagnosis of Aphasia*. Some common household objects are needed for administering the test. Record sheets may be purchased separately.

Administration
The test is divided into five sections:

(1) auditory disturbances
(2) visual and reading disturbances
(3) speech and language disturbances
(4) visual motor and writing disturbances
(5) disturbances of numerical relations and arithmetic processes.

Test items include picture, word and letter recognition; understanding sentences and following directions; reading; imitation of oral movements; naming pictures; copying letters and words; writing; and solving numerical problems. Tests are included at varying levels of difficulty and the results are a summary of scores in each of the five areas outlined above. This information may then be used for setting goals for therapy and may help in the evaluation of progress. Clinical ratings are given which indicate the client's functional competence in the areas of comprehension and expression of the spoken and written word. Normative data are provided through various studies in the Monograph. These are based on aphasic and non-aphasic subjects.

Shortened Form of the Minnesota Test for Differential Diagnosis of Aphasia (1973)

Authors
J. Thompson and
P. Enderby

Age range
Adults with acquired language disorders

Time taken
It is not a timed assessment

Publisher/Distributor
Speech Therapy Department,
Frenchay Hospital

Aims/Purpose
This shortened version of Schuell's Test (see page 95) aims to provide a comprehensive assessment of aphasia as a basis for planning treatment.

Materials
An instruction manual, score sheets, Aphasia Test Result Forms, and forms for two reading subtests are provided.

Administration
The test uses the graphic material and parts of the instruction manual supplied with the full-length Schuell Test (see page 95) and the British Amendments compiled by Davies and Grunwell in 1973 (available separately*). The assessment is divided into five sections:
(1) auditory disturbances
(2) visual and reading disturbances
(3) speech and language disturbances
(4) visuomotor and writing disturbances
(5) disturbances of numerical relations and arithmetic processes.

Each section contains a number of subtests, each of which

is made up of five stimulus items. The majority of the scoring is on a correct/error basis but a few items are scored on a clearly defined 5-point scale, according to the patient's performance. All correct items are noted and on completion of the assessment, the scores are transferred onto the Aphasia Test Result Form, giving a graphic representation of performance. Patient's performance may also be expressed in terms of its rank in the aphasic population.

*British Amendments available from: School of Speech Pathology, Leicester.

Contributions to Neuropsychological Assessment (1983)

Authors
A.L. Benton,
K. Hamsher,
N. Varney and
O. Spreen

Age range
Variable, no specific age

Time taken
This will vary according to which tests are used; none are timed

Publisher/Distributor
NFER-Nelson

Aims/Purpose
This package of 11 tests has been developed over a period of 20 years in order to assess patients over a wide range of neuropsychological functions.

Materials
A manual which includes administration and normative data for all tests. Record forms, scoring forms and additional materials required for each test may be purchased separately.

Administration
There are 11 tests.
1. *Temporal orientation*: this assesses the accuracy of a patient's temporal orientation.
2. *Right–left orientation*: a 20-item test to assess spatial thinking.
3. *Serial digit learning*: a standardised test which may be used to help differential diagnosis between brain-diseased and normal patients, as well as to assess short-term memory.
4. *Facial recognition*: a standardised procedure to assess objectively the capacity to identify and discriminate between photographs of unfamiliar people.
5. *Judgement of line orientation*: this may help to indicate brain disease, particularly in the right hemisphere.
6. *Visual form discrimination*: a short assessment procedure using complex visual forms.
7. *Tactile form perception*: this may be used to assess non-verbal tactile information processing with patients who have failed on tactile object naming and matching tasks.

8. *Finger localisation:* a non-verbal 60 item test assessing three different forms of defective finger recognition.
9. *Phoneme discrimination:* a brief screening procedure.
10. *Three-dimensional block construction:* a standardised test to evaluate three-dimensional constructional praxis.
11. *Motor impersistence:* this assesses patients' ability to sustain a movement which they were able to initiate on command.

All normative data were collated in the USA.

The Neurosensory Centre Comprehensive Examination for Aphasia (1991)

Authors
O. Spreen and A.L Benton

Age range
Normative data are available for aphasic adults, non-aphasic brain-damaged clients, normal adults and children from 6 to 13 years

Time taken
It is untimed

Publisher/Distributor
Neuro Psychology Laboratories, University of Victoria, Canada

Also described in Spreen, O. and Strauss, E. (1991) *Compendium of Neuropsychological Tests.* New York: OUP.

(This was revised and re-standardised in 1977 and replaces the *Spreen–Benton Aphasia Tests (1969).*)

Aims/Purpose
These tests were developed to assess language functions in aphasic patients: understanding; production; retention of verbal materials; reading and writing.

Materials
A manual, answer sheets and profile forms are available; 24 test objects and other materials are to be provided by the tester.

Administration
There are 20 language tests and 4 'control' tests of visual and tactile function. The latter are designed to detect the presence of visual and tactile deficits which might affect performance on the language tests; they include tests of form perception and tactile–visual matching of objects. The language tests include naming of objects, description of use, sentence and digit repetition, sentence construction, identification by sentence (using the *Token Test* material), oral reading, reading comprehension, writing and articulation tests. The raw scores for each test can be corrected for the age and educational level of the patient and translated into a percentile. Thus, both overall performance level and specific areas of deficit can easily be seen.

Porch Index of Communicative Ability (PICA) (1971)

Author
B.E. Porch

Age range
Adults with aphasia

Time taken
It is not timed, but takes approximately 1 hour

Publisher
Consulting Psychologists Press, USA

Distributor
Oxford Psychologists Press

Aims/Purpose
PICA aims to provide a standardised test battery which sensitively and reliably quantifies the patient's ability to communicate. There is particular emphasis on the provision of a reliable scoring system.

Materials
Text, administrative manual, test booklet, test objects, stimulus cards and score sheets are provided in a carrying case. A tape-recorder is useful.

Administration
The various subtests are '...not dissimilar to those usually found in aphasia tests'. At various levels of complexity, the patient is required to listen, speak, read, write, feel and gesture. There are twelve tests requiring a verbal/gestural response and six requiring a written/drawn response. Scoring is based upon five dimensions: accuracy, responsiveness, completeness, promptness and efficiency. These dimensions have been used to provide 16 scoring categories and each item of each subtest is scored, using one of these categories. An overall score can be obtained giving a view of the patient's general communicative ability. Three modality response levels – gestural, verbal and graphic – can also be estimated and a profile plotted for ease of comparison of the three levels. It has been standardised in the USA.

(In order to gain maximum benefit from use, clinicians are urged to attend training workshops, or to obtain training from an experienced user. Information regarding training from: PICA Workshops.)

Psycholinguistic Assessments of Language Processing in Aphasia (PALPA) (1992)

Authors
J. Kay, R. Lesser and M. Coltheart

Aims/Purpose
PALPA aims to enable users to investigate both impaired and intact abilities of the adult with aphasia. The resulting detailed profile may be useful as a clinical instrument and as a research tool.

Age range
Adults with acquired aphasia

Time taken
The tests are not timed

Publisher/Distributor
Laurence Erlbaum Associates

Materials
The package consists of a box containing spirally bound sets of tests and instructions, as well as master sheets of profiles, score sheets and record forms which may be photocopied.

Administration
There are approximately 60 tests of components of language structure. These include: orthography, phonology, word and picture semantics, morphology and syntax. They make use of procedures such as lexical decision, repetition and picture naming and are designed to access spoken and written input and output modalities. The user may select language tasks which are appropriate to investigate the abilities and disabilities of each individual client. Comprehensive guidelines are included to help the user in this selection task, as well as details regarding how and why each test was constructed. The responses to the tests are recorded on the sheets provided, and the resulting profile may be interpreted within current cognitive models of language in order to facilitate diagnosis and intervention planning.

The Right Hemisphere Language Battery (1989)

Author
K.L. Bryan

Age range
Not specified, but it is suitable for neurologically impaired adults

Time taken
About 30 minutes is required for administration of the battery

Publisher
Far Communications

Distributors
Far Communications
Winslow Press

Aims/Purpose
The battery was designed primarily to assess right hemisphere-damaged patients for the presence of language disorders that are associated with the disruption of right hemisphere functioning. A further clinical use for the battery is in determining whether right hemisphere language skills are preserved in left hemisphere-damaged aphasics. This is of potential value in determining whether therapy techniques which aim to increase right hemisphere participation are appropriate for a particular patient.

Materials
The battery consists of a test manual which summarises the types of language disruption that can occur after right hemisphere damage, and outlines the development of the tests as well as their usage. Examples of patient data are also included in the manual. Six sets of test materials are included with all the necessary scoring sheets and summary profile sheets. The master copies of these sheets can be photocopied.

Administration
The battery consists of six tests:
(1) metaphor picture test
(2) written metaphor test
(3) comprehension of inferred meaning
(4) appreciation of humour
(5) lexical–semantic test
(6) comprehension of inferred meaning.

In addition a discourse analysis is made by rating a series of discourse parameters. The raw scores are converted into relative T scores for each test (using a simple conversion table provided in the test manual) and are then recorded on the patient's profile sheet. This allows comparison of scores across the tests as well as a judgement of the patient's overall performance.

The Token Test (1962)

Authors
E. de Renzi and
L.A. Vignolo

Age range
Adult aphasic patients

Time taken
It is not a timed test

Publisher
The Test appears in: de Renzi, E. and Vignolo, L.A. (1962) The Token Test: A sensitive test to detect receptive disturbances in aphasics. *Brain*, 85, pp. 665–678

Aims/Purpose
This test aims 'to detect receptive disturbances in aphasics', i.e. particular slight receptive difficulties which may not be easily apparent in normal conversation. The authors' aim was to produce a test with short commands which might be easy for the patient to memorise, but which would make considerable demands on comprehension.

Materials
The Test is written up in an article. Materials required are: 20 tokens (to be made by the tester) of two different shapes, two different sizes and five different colours.

Administration
The instructions are divided into five sections of commands which become progressively linguistically complex. Simple manual responses are required. Analysis of the errors made may reveal particular receptive problems.

Revised Token Test (1978)

Authors
M.M. McNeil and
T.E. Prescott

Age range
Adults from 20 to 80 years

Time taken
Each subtest is timed

Publisher
PRO-ED, USA

Distributors
Taskmaster Ltd
Winslow Press

[This is a revised version of *The Token Test* (1962) by E. de Renzi and L.A. Vignolo – see page 101.]

Aims/Purpose
The Revised Token Test aims to assess the central auditory system in adults using a behavioural method. It was designed as a clinical as well as a research tool. Therefore it aims to be differentially diagnostic, capable of finite descriptions of auditory disorders and sensitive to mild dysfunction, as well as to patient change.

Materials
There are 24 tokens of differing colours, sizes and shapes. There is a test manual, administration manual, subtest scoring forms and profile forms, all in a sturdy box.

Administration
The profile forms are used to chart the patient's performance in terms of subtest response, command response and performance change. There are 10 subtests of increasing complexity. The basic structure of the test is the same as the 1962 version. However, each response is scored on a 15-point system, acknowledging such features as completeness, repetition and cueing. A detailed description of the system is given in the Test Manual. The test has been standardised on a normal population and patients with right hemisphere damage (non-aphasic). Percentile ranks are given for normal, right and left hemisphere brain-damaged adults for each of the 10 subtests and for overall performance.

The Western Aphasia Battery (WAB) (1982)

Author
A. Kertesz

Age range
Neurologically impaired adults

Aims/Purpose
It was designed to evaluate the main clinical aspects of language function in people with aphasia, and to provide the data needed to establish a prognosis for therapy. It also assesses some non-verbal skills.

Materials
The test consists of a test manual, an 18-page test booklet for recording performance, and 57 picture stimulus cards.

Time taken
It is not a timed test, and subtests may be administered on consecutive days

Publisher
Harcourt Brace Jovanovich

Distributor
The Psychological Corporation

Administration
The assessment procedure is based on the principles of modern neurolinguistics and the neuroanatomical language model. It enables the clinician to classify clients in relation to various aphasic groups. The WAB comprises eight subtests which provide assessment of:
(1) content
(2) fluency
(3) auditory comprehension
(4) repetition
(5) naming
(6) reading
(7) writing
(8) calculation.
On completion of the assessment, an Aphasia Quotient may be calculated which indicates the severity of language impairment.

APRAXIA

Apraxia Battery for Adults (ABA) (1979)

Author
B.L. Dabul

Age range
Adolescents and adults

Time taken
The six subtests take approximately 20 minutes to administer

Publisher
PRO-ED, USA

Distributors
Taskmaster Ltd
Winslow Press

Aims/Purpose
This systematic set of tasks aims to verify the presence of apraxia in the adult patient and to estimate the severity of the disorder. Re-assessment at intervals should provide information regarding improvement in function of motor speech programming.

Materials
The materials consist of a manual and score sheets packaged in a box. It is recommended that the tester has a stopwatch.

Administration
The ABA consists of six subtests:
(1) diadochokinetic rate
(2) increasing word length
(3) limb apraxia and oral apraxia
(4) latency and utterance time for polysyllabic words
(5) repeated trials test
(6) inventory of articulation characteristics of apraxia (spontaneous speech).
Examples of the scoring of the subtests are given in the manual. There is an objective scoring system. When the test is completed, the subject's scores are entered on a summary chart and the therapist is recommended to complete the checklist of apraxic features and profile score sheet.

DEGENERATIVE DISORDER

Anomalous Sentences Repetition Test (1988)

Author
D. Weeks

Age range
Adults from 55 to 90 years, or younger brain-damaged adults

Time taken
Approximately 5 minutes for each version of the test

Publisher/Distributor
NFER-Nelson

Aims/Purpose
This test enables therapists and clinicians working in a psychogeriatric or neurological setting to make a differential diagnosis between dementia and depression, and, indirectly, to assess the severity of dementia. It may also be used to assess cognitive functioning of patients suffering from organic impairment of the central nervous system.

Materials
The test consists of a soft-backed manual and record forms.

Administration
The record forms include four versions of the test, this is to facilitate re-testing. Each version consists of two practice sentences and six test sentences. It is simple to administer, requiring immediate repetition of anomalous sentences in which the syntax and/or semantics have been degraded. Raw score errors are converted to age-adjusted scores for people of 55 years of age and upwards. These may be compared with cut-off scores for patients in the 'less than 55 years' or 'more than 55 years' age groups. Analysis of the type of errors made gives important diagnostic information. As the level of language dysfunction is quantified, it enables indirectly, the assessment of the severity of dementia. The test was standardised on 98 elderly community residents, 100 depressed patients, and 100 patients with dementia.

Dysphasia/Dementia Screening Test (1984)

Author
A.M. Phillips

Age range
Adults, age unspecified

Time taken
It takes approximately 20 minutes

Aims/Purpose
The aim of this test is to help speech and language therapists make a differential diagnosis between dementia and dysphasia. It is intended for use with people with severe communication difficulties.

Materials
The kit comprises a manual and scoring booklet in a plastic wallet.

Publisher/Distributor
Ann M. Phillips

Administration
There are five sections to be scored:
(1) auditory comprehension
(2) verbal expression
(3) reading
(4) writing
(5) problem-solving.
The test is not standardised and the scoring system may be most useful as a diagnostic tool if all responses, clues given and the time taken are recorded in full.

The Kendrick Cognitive Tests for the Elderly (1985)

Author
D. Kendrick

[These replace *The Kendrick Battery for the Detection of Dementia in the Elderly* (1979) A.J. Gibson and D.C. Kendrick.]

Age range
Adults of 55 years and over

Time taken
Approximately 15 minutes

Publisher/Distributor
NFER-Nelson

Aims/Purpose
These tests have been designed to detect differences in cognitive responses between normal, depressive, pseudo-dementing or dementing adults, and by re-testing to monitor the efficacy of therapy programmes.

Materials
The materials include a manual, record forms, the Object Learning Test cards, and the Digit Copying Test pack.

Administration
The two cognitive tests are: The Object Learning Test and the Digit Copying Test. *The Object Learning Test* consists of picture cards each with different numbers of everyday objects. *The Digit Copying Test* requires the client to copy as many digits as possible within a given time. Clients may be re-tested after a period of 6 weeks so that changes of function may be detected, and the effectiveness of therapy programmes monitored. Raw scores are obtained which may be converted into age-scaled scores in the form of quotients. Cut-off scores for both tests are provided together with new normative data. There is a comprehensive bibliography.

DYSARTHRIA

Frenchay Dysarthria Assessment and Computer Differential Analysis – second edition (1983)

Author
P. Enderby

Age range
People with dysarthria, from 15 years of age to adults

Time taken
It is untimed, dependent on the patient

Publisher/Distributor
NFER-Nelson

Aims/Purpose
This test is designed to help speech and language therapists to identify dysarthria and to give a graphic profile of the dysarthric person's abilities and disabilities, so that treatment and management programmes may be planned.

Materials
An instruction manual, score sheets and scoring graph are provided. Software for computer differential analysis is also available. This is for use with APPLE IIc, II Plus and IIe computers.

Administration
The test is divided into 11 sections:
  (1) reflexes
  (2) respiration
  (3) lips
  (4) jaw
  (5) palate
  (6) laryngeal
  (7) tongue
  (8) intelligibility
  (9) rate
  (10) sensation
  (11) associated factors.

On each section the client's performance is scored by points on a scale, for a number of simple tasks such as drinking, and repeating sounds. The manual gives a definition of the performance required for each point of the scale. On completion of the assessment, a bar chart graph is shaded so that areas of difficulty may be easily identified. By using the computer interpretation package, the profile may be instantly generated from the scores entered. Normative data are reported for normal and medically diagnosed dysarthric people. Separate tables allow for comparison of individual results with those of known dysarthric groups.

Robertson Dysarthria Profile (1982)

Author
S.J. Robertson

Age range
Adults with acquired dysarthria

Time taken
It is untimed, dependent on the patient

Publisher/Distributor
Winslow Press

Aims/Purpose
This clinical assessment procedure is designed to give a profile of the dysarthric patient's abilities and disabilities irrespective of the underlying neurological aetiology. The descriptive profile may help classification and aid treatment planning, therapy and management.

Materials
Instructional manual, forms for scoring, profile summary forms and stimulus cards are provided in a folder.

Administration
The Robertson Dysarthria Profile is divided into eight sections:
(1) respiration
(2) phonation
(3) examination of facial musculature
(4) diadochokinesis
(5) reflexes
(6) articulation
(7) intelligibility
(8) prosody and rate.

Each parameter is assessed as independently as possible within each section. There are a number of tasks to be carried out by the patient and these are scored on a 5-point scale. The manual gives details of how responses should be rated. In addition, appropriate descriptive statements are selected from a multiple choice about each parameter. The final scores are transferred onto a summary profile.

DYSPHAGIA

Dysphagia Care with Acute and Long-term Patients (1990)

Author
N. O'Sullivan

Age range
Adults with acquired dysphagia

Aims/Purpose
To suggest techniques for the practical assessment of eating/feeding problems and subsequent effective treatment of these problems through teamwork.

Materials
This is a spiral-bound, 135 page book.

Time taken
Assessment depends
upon the patient

Publisher/Distributor
Fred Sammons Inc.,
USA

Administration
This source book includes current information regarding the assessment and treatment of dysphagia, including tracheostomy weaning, diet, food progression, syringe feeding, staff in-service, and suggests exercises and restorative dining programmes.

Part V

Fluency

A Component Model G.D. Riley and J. Riley	110
Assessing Communication Attitudes among Stutterers (see S24 Scale) R.L. Erickson	
Cooper Personalised Fluency Control Therapy – Revised edition E.B. Cooper and C.S. Cooper	111
Assessment and Therapy Programme for Dysfluent Children L. Rustin	111
Systematic Fluency Training for Young Children R.E. Shine	112
The Perceptions of Stuttering Inventory G. Woolf	113
S24 Scale G. Andrews and J. Cutler	113
Stuttering Intervention Programme R. Pindzola	114
Stuttering Prediction Instrument for Young Children G.D. Riley	114
Stuttering Severity Instrument for Children and Adults G.D. Riley	115

A Component Model

Authors
G.D. Riley and J. Riley

Age range
Children, approximately 3–11 years

Time taken
Two to three hours; assessment and management are on-going

Materials
A description of the model is given by the authors in the *Journal of Fluency Disorders* (1979) and in a book edited by M. Peins (1984) (see below). Subsequently, it has been more fully described in articles by the authors, and a selection of references is given below.

Administration
This approach offers a component model to the assessment and treatment of dysfluent children. Based on their research, the authors have identified nine components that seem to be significant in the development of stuttering. The components are grouped under three main headings:
(1) neurological
(2) intrapersonal
(3) interpersonal.
Components listed under these headings range from attending and oral–motor disorders, to a disruptive communicative environment and the high self-expectations of the child. The treatment and management of the child is then based on the remediation of those components which are found to be relevant in each case.

References
Riley, G.D. and Riley, J.A. (1979). A component model for diagnosing and treating children who stutter. *Journal of Fluency Disorders* **4**, 279–293.
Riley, G.D. and Riley, J.A. (1984). A component model for treating stuttering in children. In M. Peins (Ed.) *Contemporary Approaches in Stuttering Therapy*. Boston: Little, Brown & Co.
Riley, G.D. and Riley, J.A. (1982). Evaluating stuttering problems in children. *Journal of Childhood Communication Disorders* **VI** (1), 15–25.
Riley, G.D. and Riley, J.A. (1983). Evaluation as a basis for intervention. In D. Preins and R. Ingham (Eds) *Treatment of Stuttering in Early Childhood*. San Diego, CA: College-Hill.

Cooper Personalised Fluency Control Therapy – Revised edition (1985)

Authors
E.B. Cooper and C.S. Cooper

Age range
Children, from pre-school to adolescents, and adults

Time taken
The assessment is not timed as it is on-going with therapy

Publisher
DLM Teaching Resources, USA

Distributor
Taskmaster Ltd

Aims/Purpose
This is a total programme of assessment and treatment for anyone who stutters. Information and material are provided to enable parents, teachers and therapists help the stuttering person develop control of their stutter.

Materials
A carrying case contains a handbook, a book of 112 black-line masters, including Individualised Educational Program (IEP) forms, assignment/evaluation worksheets, practice and activity sheets, guides, attitude checklist, readiness inventory and fluency checklist; two assessment digest and treatment plan booklets, one for children and one for adolescents and adults; games boards and appropriate items for play.

Administration
The handbook gives detailed instructions on how to use the materials for assessment, followed by short- or long-term therapy. The programme is based on over 25 years of teaching and research. It integrates activities to deal with the affective, cognitive and behavioural aspects of the stutterer's difficulties. The approach of the programme is to give the stutterer a feeling of control, in order that fluency might follow, rather than developing an arbitrary level of fluency.

Assessment and Therapy Programme for Dysfluent Children (1987)

Author
L. Rustin

Age range
Children, mainly 7–13 years; some parts may be used with children from 2;6 to 7 years

Aims/Purpose
It aims to provide a structured assessment of the dysfluent child. It offers detailed guidance so that the results of the initial assessment may be used to set up appropriate individualised therapy programmes. It may be used with individuals, or in groups for weekly or intensive therapy.

Materials
The kit, in a plastic folder, comprises work books, task sheets and a soft-backed manual. An audio cassette is also provided, so that a tape-recorder will be required.

Time taken
It is not a timed assessment

Publisher/Distributor
NFER-Nelson

Administration
The 12-page booklet gives details of structured interviews with parents and children. These interviews enable the clinician to gather information regarding the child's fluency, socioemotional background, behaviour and environment. Detailed suggestions are then given in the manual to show how these results may be used to devise an individualised programme. The audio-cassette provides examples of therapy techniques for the clinician. Work books and task sheets are structured so that parental and familial involvement in the child's therapy programme may be encouraged. They may also be used to record and monitor progress.

Systematic Fluency Training for Young Children (1980)

Author
R.E. Shine

Age range
Children from 3 to 9 years

Time taken
It is not a timed test

Publisher
PRO-ED, USA

Distributors
Taskmaster Ltd
Winslow Press

Aims/Purpose
This pack is intended to provide a comprehensive assessment and training procedure for the direct management of young children who stutter.

Materials
A manual, picture stimulus cards, lotto games, surprise toy box, story books, record forms, and an audio-cassette, are included in a carrying case. A tape-recorder will be required.

Administration
This procedure is behaviourally based. It includes: methods of assessment, parent counselling, home programmes and environmental transfer procedures. Basic rationale and training procedures are described in the manual. The audio-cassette may be used to train the counting of stuttered words, and to provide a model of specific speech production. The programme may be individually administered.

The Perceptions of Stuttering Inventory (1967)

Author
G. Woolf

Age range
Adolescents and adults

Time taken
It is not a timed assessment

Aims/Purpose
The inventory is of use to both the client and the therapist as the aims are: to describe what the stutterer does when he/she stutters; to broaden the stutterer's understanding and definition of his/her problems, and to analyse the pattern of relationships among struggle, avoidance and expectancy. The results may then be used to help formulate appropriate goals for therapy, and evaluate progress towards these goals.

Materials
The complete inventory may be found in the article listed below.

Administration
It may be administered to a group or individually. The subjects are required to answer 60 items representing equally the stuttering parameters of struggle, avoidance and expectancy. There are 20 items for each dimension. Directions may be given orally or in written form.

Reference
Woolf, G. (1967). The assessment of stuttering as struggle, avoidance and expectancy. *British Journal of Disorders of Communication* 2, 158–171.

S24 Scale (1974)

Authors
G. Andrews and J. Cutler

Age range
Adolescents and adults

Time taken
It is not a timed assessment

Aims/Purpose
This is a questionnaire, designed to measure the stutterer's attitude to interpersonal communication.

Materials
It is a single page questionnaire.

Administration
The S24 Scale has been adapted from the article: Erickson, R.L. (1969). Assessing communication attitudes among stutterers. *Journal of Speech and Hearing Research* 12, 711–724. There is an inventory of 24 items requiring a true or false response. It may be administered in written form or questions and answers may be given verbally. This revised scale is more suited to repeated administration. There is

some evidence to suggest that a low S24 score after treatment might indicate favourable long-term outcome.

Reference
Andrews, G. and Cutler, J. (1974). Stuttering therapy: The relation between changes in symptom level and attitudes. *Journal of Speech and Hearing Disorders* **39**, 313–319.

Stuttering Intervention Programme (1987)

Author
R. Pindzola

Age range
Children from 3 to 9 years

Time taken
This is an ongoing assessment and programme

Publisher/Distributor
Modern Education Corporation, USA

Aims/Purpose
The programme aims to provide a package for fluency management in children from pre-school to school age, and to offer direct intervention strategies for the incipient stutterer.

Materials
The package consists of a folder containing a manual and assessment forms, which include parental interview forms.

Administration
The assessment and programme consists of several sections. There are *Assessment Procedures* which may be used as a screening test or a more in-depth test of dysfluency; *Guidelines for Counselling and Training*; a *Direct Fluency Management Program* which fosters fluency through an operant conditioning paradigm, enhances fluency through altered physiological speaking processes and decreases the possibility of fluency disruption through linguistic manipulation; *Formats for Individual Educational Programs* and *Information Packages for Teachers/Schools*.

Stuttering Prediction Instrument for Young Children (1981)

Author
G.D. Riley

Age range
Children from 3 to 8 years

Aims/Purpose
The aim of this assessment is to provide information on the type and severity of the dysfluency, to discern the presence of environmental influences, and to help in the decision as to whether the dysfluency is developmental. It is also designed to be used for research purposes.

Time taken
It is not a timed assessment

Publisher
PRO-ED, USA

Distributors
Taskmaster Ltd
Winslow Press

Materials
There is a manual, test forms and stimulus materials.

Administration
The stimulus materials consist of five black and white line drawings of everyday situations which are used as topics for conversation. Information is also obtained from parents or carers. The assessment is divided into five sections: a case history; parents' reactions; and analysis of part-word repetitions, prolongations and frequency of stuttering behaviour. There is a detailed but simple scoring system which provides percentiles and a severity rating. The assessment provides a basis for treatment planning. Norms have been established on children from the USA and validity was tested by comparing the scores obtained with scores on the Stuttering Severity Instrument (see below).

Stuttering Severity Instrument for Children and Adults (1980)

Author
G.D. Riley

Age range
Children and adults

Time taken
It is not a timed assessment

Publisher
PRO-ED, USA

Distributors
Taskmaster Ltd
Winslow Press

Aims/Purpose
The aim of this assessment is to provide an objective instrument to describe the severity of stuttering behaviour. It is designed for clinical and research use.

Materials
The test consists of a firm spirally bound manual and test forms which are in a carrying case. Stimulus materials, such as pictorial sequences and written paragraphs appropriate for different levels of reading ability, are included in the manual.

Administration
Three parameters are used for describing stuttering: frequency of repetition and prolongation of sounds and syllables, estimated duration of the longest blocks or stuttering occurrences, and observable visual and audible associated physical behaviours. The test form is divided into four major areas:
(1) frequency
(2) duration
(3) physical concomitants
(4) severity conversion tables for children and adults.
It yields a single numerical representation of severity within a range of 0–45. The assessment was standardised on children and adults in the USA.

APPENDIX I: Publishers/Distributors

Dr Janet Mackenzie Beck, Queen Margaret College, Clerwood Drive, Edinburgh
Dr D. Bishop, Department of Psychology, University of Manchester, Oxford Road, Manchester M13 9PL. Tel: 061-275-2557. Fax: 061-275-2588
Blissymbolics Communications (UK) Resource Centre, Thomas House, Cardiff Institute of Higher Education, Cyncoed Road, Cyncoed, Cardiff. Tel: 0222-757826
Camp Ltd, Northgate House, Staple Gardens, Winchester, Hampshire, SO23 8ST. Tel: 0962-55248. Fax: 0962-855636
Centre for Audiology, Education of the Deaf, and Speech Pathology, University of Manchester, Oxford Road, Manchester M13 9PL
Child Development Research Unit, (The Secretary), University of Nottingham, University Park, Nottingham, NG7 2RD. Tel: 0602-484848. Fax: 0602-590339
Churchill Livingstone (see Longmans)
Communication Skill Builders (Therapy Skill Builders), 3830 E Bellevue, PO Box 42050, Tucson, Arizona 85733, USA
Consulting Psychologists Press Inc., 3803 E Bayshore Road, PO Box 10096, Palo Alto, CA 94303, USA
Professor David Crystal, PO Box 5, Holyhead, Gwynedd LL65 1RG. Tel: 0407-2764
DLM Teaching Resources, One DLM Park, Allen, Texas, 75002, USA
Educational Center, Coop Care Building, 14th Floor, New York University Medical Center, 530 First Ave, New York, NY 10016, USA
Educational Evaluation Enterprises, Awre, Newnham, Glos GL14 1ET. Tel: 0594-510503
Laurence Erlbaum Associates, 27 Church Road, Hove, East Sussex, BN3 2FA. Tel: 0273-207411
Far Communications, 5 Harcourt Estate, Kibworth, Leicestershire, LE8 0NE. Tel: 0533-796166
Forum Consultancy, 1/9 St Mark's Road, London W11
Harcourt Brace Jovanovich (see The Psychological Corporation)
Heinemann Educational Books Ltd, Inspection Copy Department, Sanders Lodge Estate, Rushden, Northants NN10 9BR. Tel: 0933-58521
Hodder and Stoughton Publishers, Mill Road, Dunton Green, Sevenoaks, Kent TN13 2YA. Tel: 0732-450111. Fax: 0732-460134
IMAGINART Communication Products, 307 Arizona St, Bisbee, AZ 85603 USA. Fax: 602-432-5134
Professor John Laver, Centre for Speech Technology, University of Edinburgh, South Bridge, Edinburgh
LDA, Duke St, Wisbech, Cambs PE13 2AE. Tel: 0945-63441. Fax: 0945-587361
Lea and Febiger, PO Box 8068-607, Philadelphia, PA 19177, USA. Fax: 215-251-2229
Linguisystems Inc., 3100 4th Avenue, PO Box 747, East Moline, Illinois 61244, USA
Longman Group UK Ltd, PO Box 77, Harlow, Essex CM19 5BQ. Tel: 0279-429655. Fax: 0279-431067
Macmillan Education, Houndmills, Basingstoke, Hants RG21 2XS. Tel: 0256-29242. Fax: 0256-479476
Mark Masidlover, Chief Educational Psychologist, Derbyshire Education Authority, Grosvenor Road, Ripley DE5 3JE
MENCAP Bookshop, 123 Golden Lane, London EC1Y 0RT. Tel: 071-454 0454
Modern Education Corporation, PO Box 721, Tulsa, Oklahoma, 74101, USA
NFER-Nelson, Darville House, 2 Oxford Road East, Windsor, Berks SL4 1DF. Tel: 0753 858961. Fax: 0753-856830
Neuropsychology Laboratories, Department of Psychology, University of Victoria, British Columbia, Canada V8W 3P5 Fax: 604-721-8929
New York University Medical Center, Institute of Rehabilitation Medicine, 400 East 34th Street, New York, NY 10016, USA

Oxford Psychologists Press, Lambourne House, 311–321 Banbury Road, Oxford, OX2 7JH. Tel: 0865-510203. Fax: 0865-310368
Ann M. Phillips, Practice Manager, 4 St Peter's Place, Brighton BN1 4SA. Tel: 0273 681012
PICA Workshops, 713 Parkland Circle, SE, Albuquerque, NM 87108, USA
J.A. Preston Corporation, 60 Page Road, Clifton, New Jersey, NJ 07012, USA
PRO-ED, 8700 Shoal Creek Boulevard, Austin, Texas 78758-9965, USA. Fax: 512-451-8542
The Psychological Corporation, Foots Cray High St, Sidcup, Kent DA14 5HP. Tel: 081-300 3322. Fax: 081-309 0807
C.E. Renfrew, 2A North Place, Old Headington, Oxford OX3 9HX
Fred Sammons Inc., 145 Tower Drive, Burr Ridge, IL 60521, USA. Fax: 708-325-4602
SEFA (Publications) Ltd, The Globe, 4 Great William St, Stratford-upon-Avon, Warks
Ms Christina Shewell, National Hospital's College of Speech Sciences, Chandler House, 2 Wakefield St, London WC1N 1PG
School of Speech Pathology, Scraptoft Campus, Scraptoft, Leicester Polytechnic, Leicester LE7 9SU
Special Education Resource Centre, Anson Road, Manchester 14
Speech Therapy Department, Frenchay Hospital, Bristol BS16 1LE. Tel: 0272-701212, ext. 2255/2296
Speech Therapy Department, Nuffield Hearing and Speech Centre, Royal National Throat, Nose and Ear Hospital, Gray's Inn Rd, London WC1X 8DA. Tel: 071-837 8855
Speech Profiles, c/o The Old Post Office, Newland, Nr Coleford, Glos GL16 8NP
STASS Publications, 44 North Road, Ponteland, Northumberland NE20 9UR. Tel: 0661-22316
Taskmaster Ltd, Morris Road, Leicester LE2 6BR. Tel: 0533-704286. Fax: 0533-706992
Therapy Skill Builders (see Communication Skill Builders)
Western Psychological Services, 12031 Wilshire Boulevard, Los Angeles, California 90025, USA. Fax: 213-478-7838
Whurr Publishers, 19B Compton Terrace, London N1 2UN. Tel: 071-359 5979. Fax: 071-226 5290
Williams and Wilkins, The Broadway Centre, 2–6 Fulham Broadway, London SW6 1AA. Tel: 071-385 2357. Fax: 071-385 2922
Winslow Press, Telford Road, Bicester, Oxon OX6 0TS. Tel: 0869-244733. Fax: 0869-320040
Dr Sheila Wirz, National Hospital's College of Speech Sciences, Chandler House, 2 Wakefield St, London WC1N 1PG

APPENDIX II: Some tests which are out of print

Articulation Attainment Test by C.E. Renfrew
Developmental Guide to Comprehension of Grammar by M. Berry (USA)
Inventory for the Assessment of Laryngectomy Rehabilitation by La Borwit, C.C. Publications
Language Imitation Test by P. Berry and P. Mittler, NFER-Nelson
Picture Pointing Auditory Discrimination Test by C.E. Renfrew

Some tests which are in press, due to be published in 1992, which may be of interest to speech and language therapists

Nuffield Centre Dyspraxia Programme, The Speech Therapy Department, Nuffield Hearing and Speech Centre: a new edition of this programme (see page 10 for first edition) was due for publication at the end of 1991. This incorporates a new assessment procedure and some changes in the picture stimulus material. A 'conversion kit' will be available for use with the first edition.

Social Use of Language Programme by W. Rinaldi, NFER-Nelson: a programme for assessing and developing social use of language in real-life settings, for adolescents and adults with hearing impairment, speech and language difficulties, and/or people with learning difficulties.

Author Index

Aarons, M., 72
Ainley, M., 52, 62
Anderson, J., 67
Andrews, G., 113
Anthony, A., 8
Armstrong, S., 52, 62

Bankson, N.W., 36
Barber, M., 72
Barton, L., 72
Bate, M., 25
Beech, 55
Bellman, M., 23
Benton, A.L., 97, 98
Bishop, D.V.M., 56
Blakeley, R.W., 8
Blodgett, E.G., 46
Boder, E., 66
Boehm, A.E., 19
Bogle, D., 8
Bolton, S., 77
Boone, D., 2
Bracken, B.A., 19
Bradley, L., 71
Brimer, M.A., 42
Brown, L.H., 76
Brown, V.L., 35
Bryan, K.L., 100
Bzoch, K., 50

Cameron, R.J., 26
Carrow-Woolfolk, E., 31, 36, 39
Cash, J., 23
Christophers, U., 69
Claydon, J., 71
Collins, L., 72
Coltheart, M., 99
Cooper, C.S., 111
Cooper, E.B., 46, 111
Costello, A., 21
Coupe, J., 72
Crystal, D., 43
Cutler, J., 113

Dabul, B., 103
Dashiell, S.E., 77
Dean, E., 59, 92
de la Mare, M., 68, 70
de Renzi, E., 101
Dewart, H., 62
DiSimoni, F., 56
Duncan, D., 34
Dunn, L.M., 38
Dunn, L.M., 38, 42
Dunn Klein, M., 79

Dunst, C.J., 81

Eisenson, J., 91
Enderby, P., 93, 96, 106
Erickson, R.L., 113
Evans, S., 90
Evans Morris, S., 28, 79

Fletcher, P., 43
Fristoe, M., 9, 31
Frostig, M., 82

Garman, M., 43
German, D.J., 57, 58
Gibbs, D., 33, 34
Gittens, T., 72
Goldman, R., 9, 31
Goldsworthy, C.L., 48
Goodenough, F.L., 20
Goodglass, H., 89–90
Grunwell, P., 60, 61
Gunzburg, H.C., 64
Gutfreund, M., 37

Hammill, D.D., 35, 41, 45
Hamsher, K., 97
Harris, D.B., 20
Harrison, M., 37
Hickson, F.S., 32
Hill, A., 59
Hitchings, A., 78
Hobsbaum, A., 34
Holland, A., 91
Howell, J., 59
Hresko, W.H., 41
Huntley, M., 51

Ingram, T.T.S., 8

Jarrico, S., 66
Jeffree, D.M., 25
Jones, B.W., 54
Jones, M., 73
Jones, S., 77

Kaplan, E., 89–90
Kay, J., 99
Keens, A., 76
Kendrick, D., 105
Kertesz, A., 102
Kiernan, C., 73, 80
Kirk, S., 43
Kirk, W., 43
Knowles, W., 75

Larsen, S., 35
Laver, J., 3
League, R., 50
Lee Wiederholt, J., 35
Lesser, R., 99
Levy, D., 72
Locke, A., 47, 55
Lowe, M., 21

Mackenzie, J., 3
McCarthy, J., 43
McConkey, R., 25
McGuire, J., 27
McIsaac, M.W., 8
McKenna, P., 95
McLeod, J., 67
McNeill, M.M., 102
Masidlover, M., 175
Mittler, P., 34
Mogford, K., 75
Mohammed Whittaker, H., 33
Morency, A., 30
Morgan Barry, R., 29
Murphy, D., 72

Neale, M.D., 69
Nelson, H.E., 69
Newcomer, P.L., 45
Newton, M., 66

O'Sullivan, N., 107

Phillips, A.M., 104
Pindzola, R., 114
Pintilie, D., 38
Pond, R.E., 49
Porch, B.E., 48, 99
Power, D.J., 54
Prescott, T.E., 102

Quigley, S.P., 54

Raven, J.C., 21
Reid, B., 80
Reid, D.K., 41
Renfrew, C.E., 35, 38, 59
Reynell, J.K., 51, 52
Reynolds, W.M., 30
Richman, N., 27
Riley, G.D., 110, 114, 115
Riley, J., 110
Robertson, S.J., 107
Ruscello, D.M., 10
Rustin, L., 111

St Louis, K.O., 10
Sarno, M.T., 94
Saund, S., 34
Schuell, H., 95
Secord, W., 40, 44, 48
Semell, E., 40
Sheridan, M., 33, 53, 82
Shine, R., 112
Shulman, B.B., 63
Singh Noor, N., 33
Skinner, C., 92
Smith, M., 25
Spence, R., 78
Spence, S., 65
Spreen, O., 97, 98
Steiner, V.G., 49
Steinkamp, M.W., 54
Summers, S., 62

Thompson, J., 96
Thomson, M., 66
Thorum, A.R., 42

Unwin, D., 67

van der Gaag, A., 74
Varney, N., 97
Vignolo, L.A., 101
Vincent, D., 68, 70, 71

Wade, D., 93
Warrington, E., 95
Waters, D., 59
Weeks, D., 104
Weiner, F.F., 61
Weintraub, S., 90
Wells, G., 37
Weschler, D., 22
Wepman, J.M., 30
Wheldall, K., 34
Whetton, C., 38, 69
White, M., 26
Whitehouse, J., 24
Whurr, R., 88, 90
Wiig, E.H., 40, 44, 46
Wilson, D.K., 3
Wirz, S.L., 92
Wood, V., 93
Woodcock, R., 31
Woolf, G., 113

Zimmerman, I.L., 49
Zinkin, P., 52

Title Index

Action Picture Test, 35
Affective Communication Assessment, 72
Analysis of the Language of Learning, 46
Anomalous Sentences Repetition Test, 104
An Aphasia Screening Test, 88
Apraxia Battery for Adults, 103
The Assessment of Aphasia and Related Disorders, see The Boston Diagnostic Aphasia Examination
Assessing Communication Attitudes among Stutterers, see S24 Scale
Assessing Reading Difficulties, 71
Assessment in Nursery Education, 25
Assessment and Therapy Programme for Dysfluent Children, 111
The Aston Index, 66
Auditory Discrimination and Attention Test, 29
Auditory Memory Span Test, 30

Bankson Language Test, 36
Behaviour Assessment Battery, 73
The Boder Test of Reading–Spelling Patterns, 66
Boehm Test of Basic Concepts, 19
The Boone Voice Program for Adults, 2
The Boone Voice Program for Children, 2
The Boston Diagnostic Aphasia Examination, 89
The Boston Naming Test, 90
Bracken Basic Concept Scale, 19
Bristol Language Development Scales, 37
British Picture Vocabulary Scale, 38
The Buffalo III Voice Profile Scheme, 3
The Bus Story, 38

Carrow Auditory–Visual Abilities Test, 31
Carrow Elicited Language Inventory, 39
The Children's Aphasia Screening Test, 90
A Clinical and Educational Manual for use with the Uzgiris and Hunt Scales of Infant Psychological Development, 81
Clinical Evaluation of Language Fundamentals, 40
Clinical Language Intervention Programme, 40
The Communication Assessment Profile for Adults with a Mental Handicap, 74
The Communication Schedule, 75
Communicative Abilities in Daily Living, 91
A Component Model, 110
Contributions to Neuropsychological Assessment, 97
Cooper Personalised Fluency Control Therapy, 111

The Derbyshire Language Scheme, 75
Developmental Test of Visual Perception, 82
Diagnostic Spelling Test, 71
Dysphagia Care with Acute and Long-term Patients, 107
Dysphasia/Dementia Screening Test, 104

Edinburgh Articulation Test, 8
ENABLE – Encouraging a Natural and Better Life Experience, 76
English Picture Vocabulary Test, 42
Examining for Aphasia, 91

Frenchay Aphasia Screening Test, 93
Frenchay Dysarthria Assessment and Computer Differential Analysis, 106
Fullerton Language Test for Adolescents, 42
Functional Communication Profile, 94

GAP Reading Comprehension Test, 67
GAPADOL Reading Comprehension Test, 67
Goldman–Fristoe Test of Articulation, 9
Goldman–Fristoe–Woodcock Auditory Skills Test Battery, 31
Goodenough–Harris Drawing Test, 20
Graded Naming Test, 95

Illinois Test of Psycholinguistic Abilities, 43
Intecom, 77
The Interactive Checklist for Augmentative Communication, 78
Is this Autism?, 73

The Kendrick Cognitive Tests for the Elderly, 105

Language Assessment Remediation and Screening Procedure, 44
Let's Talk – Inventory for Adolescents, 46
Let's Talk – Inventory for Children, 47
Living Language, 47
London Reading Test, 67

Macmillan Individual Reading Analysis, 68
The Manchester Picture Test, 32
Metaphon Resource Pack, 59
Minnesota Test for Differential Diagnosis of Aphasia, 95
The Mossford Assessment Chart for the Physically Handicapped, 24
Multilevel Informal Language Inventory, 48

National Adult Reading Test, 69
Neale Analysis of Reading Ability, 69
The Neurosensory Centre Comprehensive Examination for Aphasia, 98
New Macmillan Reading Analysis, 70
Nuffield Centre Dyspraxia Programme, 10

Oral Speech Mechanism Screening Examination, 10

PACS Pictures: Language Elicitation Materials, 60
The Perceptions of Stuttering Inventory, 113

Personal Communication Plan, 78
Phonological Assessment of Child Speech, 61
Phonological Process Analysis, 61
PIP Developmental Charts, 25
Porch Index of Communicative Ability, 99
Porch Index of Communicative Ability in Children, 48
The Portage Early Education Programme, 26
Pragmatics Profile of Early Communication Skills, 62
Pre-feeding Skills, 79
Pre-school Behaviour Checklist, 27
Pre-school Language Scale, 49
Pre-speech Assessment Scale, 28
Pre-symbol Assessment, 80
Pre-verbal Communication Schedule, 80
Progress Assessment Charts of Social and Personal Development, 64
Psycholinguistic Assessments of Language Processing in Aphasia, 99

Raven's Progressive Matrices and Vocabulary Scales, 21
Receptive–Expressive Emergent Language Scale, 50
Revised Edinburgh Functional Communication Profile, 92
Revised Token Test, 102
Reynell Developmental Language Scales, 51
Reynell–Zinkin Scales for Young Visually Handicapped Children, 52
The Right Hemisphere Language Battery, 100
Robertson Dysarthria Profile, 107

S24 Scale, 113
Sandwell Bilingual Screening Assessment, 33
The Schedule of Growing Skills, 23
Screening Test for Developmental Apraxia of Speech, 8
Sentence Comprehension Test: Revised and Panjabi editions, 34

Shortened Form of the Minnesota Test for Differential Diagnosis of Aphasia, 96
Social Skills Training with Children and Adolescents, 65
South Tyneside Assessment of Phonology, 62
South Tyneside Assessment of Syntactic Structures, 52
Stuttering Intervention Programme, 114
Stuttering Prediction Instrument for Young Children, 114
Stuttering Severity Instrument for Children and Adults, 115
Stycar Hearing Tests, 33
Stycar Language Tests, 53
Stycar Vision Tests, 82
Symbolic Play Test, 21
Systematic Fluency Training for Young Children, 112

Teaching Talking, 55
Test of Adolescent Language – 2, 35
Test for Auditory Comprehension of Language, 36
Test of Early Language Development, 41
Test of Language Competence, 44
Test of Language Development – 2, 45
Test of Pragmatic Skills, 63
The Test of Syntactic Abilities, 54
Test of Word Finding, 57
Test of Word Finding in Discourse, 58
The Token Test, 101
The Token Test for Children, 56
TROG – Test for Reception of Grammar, 56

The Vocal Profiles Analysis Scheme, 4

Wechsler Memory Scale, 22
Wepman's Auditory Discrimination Test, 30
The Western Aphasia Battery, 102
Word-Finding Vocabulary Scale, 59